CONTENTS

INTRODUCTION

The Keto Diet Explained...

The ketogenic diet stands out among popular regimens – unlike many other diets, it is straightforward and easy to follow. Simply put, it involves cutting your carb intake and replacing these carbs with large amounts of fat. Food containing a high carb content causes your body to produce both insulin and glucose.

• Glucose – is a simple sugar that plays a major role in converting and using the energy we get from food, namely carbohydrates, to fuel our body.

• Insulin – is a hormone produced by the pancreas that carries glucose through our bloodstream to our cells.

Glucose is our primary source of energy. This means that most of the time, excess fat gets stored away, unused. Often, when people are unsure whether or not the ketogenic diet is for them, they try a high-carbohydrate diet first. We've been taught since elementary school that carbs are our number-one source of energy, and while this may be true, carbs do not come without their drawbacks. The keto diet eliminates these problems by substituting carbs with fats. Let's clear some things up first. There are the four types of ketogenic diet:

• Standard Ketogenic Diet (SKD) – This type of keto diet is the most popular and comes highly recommended from nutritionists. For the SKD, you'll consume a high proportion of fat (roughly 75% of your caloric intake) and keep your protein intake moderate (20%). That last 5% will be reserved for carbs.

• High-Protein Ketogenic Diet – Just as you might expect, this type of keto diet involves eating high volumes of protein. Your calorie intake should amount to roughly 60% fat, 35% protein and 5% carbohydrates.

• Targeted Ketogenic Diet (TKD) – This one gives you more wiggle-room in terms of your carb intake. It's a good fit for athletes, who use up their glycogen reserves quickly.

• Cyclical Ketogenic Diet (CKD) – With the CKD, your diet will change from day to day. Usually this means dedicating two days a week to high carb consumption, with the other five being strictly ketogenic.

While the standard ketogenic diet is a favorite among beginners, it is important to also consider the other three as one of them may be better suited to your body type, personal goals, and lifestyle. That being said, I always recommend starting with the SKD to test the water and paying close attention to how your body adapts to the new diet, as well as any possible side effects you might experience. Many of my students get great results with the standard diet right off the bat – some of them even exceed my expectations!

Macros

The term 'macro' is an abbreviation of the word 'macronutrient', which in turn refers to 'the big three' – carbohydrates, proteins, and fats. Use the macro calculator to find out your personal daily intake requirements. Fats cause a minute amount of glucose to be released when our bodies convert triglycerides; as a result, it is said that fats are 90% ketogenic and 10% anti-ketogenic. Proteins are roughly 45% ketogenic and 55% anti-ketogenic, because half of the proteins we consume are converted to glucose in the body, which leads to a rise in insulin. Carbs are 100% anti-ketogenic – they are the main culprits in spiking our insulin and blood glucose levels. So what does this mean? Simply put, carbs and protein are our main obstacles when trying to reach ketosis. It is therefore vital to understand the metabolic pathways through which they are converted into energy after they are ingested.

At this point you might be wondering what kind of toll such a significant change to your diet is going to take on how you feel, especially if you are used to consuming higher amounts of carbohydrates. Your body may have built up a stock of carbohydrate-active enzymes, and therefore might not be well-equipped to break down and store large volumes of fat, or to deal with a sudden shortage of glucose. As a result, your body has to produce an entirely new supply of enzymes. After an adjustment period, your body will naturally begin to use your reserves of glucose, stored in the liver and muscles, for energy. This can lead to lethargy and sluggishness.

Many people cite dizziness, headaches and irritability as early side effects of the keto diet, particularly during the first seven days. This is due to the depletion of electrolytes from your system, which is, of course, another reason to drink plenty of fluids and replenish your sodium levels. As a matter of fact, since sodium helps retain water in the body, many dieticians recommend upping your salt intake significantly.

KETO HISTORY
20th century—Present

Would you believe that the keto diet dates as far back as the 1920s? In fact, it predates most other popular diets. In its initial stages the ketogenic diet was used as a treatment for epilepsy, as it was found that periods of fasting helped to minimize seizures. The keto diet was therefore a helpful and effective precursor to the various medications that were later developed to combat symptoms of epilepsy, like insulin injections. Interestingly enough, 20% to 30% of sufferers of epilepsy today still find the ketogenic diet more effective than medication. Indeed, many practitioners will still recommend it as an alternative remedy due to the additional health benefits that will be covered later in this book.

To get more specific, the endocrinologist Rollin Woodyatt found in 1921 that maintaining a ketogenic diet allows our liver to produce three water-soluble compounds:

- β-hydroxybutyrate
- acetoacetate
- acetone

These compounds are what we call ketone bodies. In the early 20th century, the American writer Bernarr Macfadden advocated fasting as a means of improving one's health and well-being. His student osteopath Hugh Conklin subsequently introduced fasting as a method of alleviating symptoms of epilepsy. This was based on Conklin's hypothesis that fasting for 18 to 25 days could completely rid the body of the toxin that causes epileptic seizures. The 'water diet' with which he prescribed his patients had outstanding results: 20% of his patients became seizure-free, while a further 50% manifested a significant improvement in their condition. Fasting therapy was soon fostered into mainstream therapy practices. In 1916, a report published in the *New York Medical Journal* revealed that one Dr McMurray had successfully treated sufferers of epilepsy with his low-calorie regimen, which was completely free of starch.

The name 'ketogenic diet' can be attributed to Dr Russell Wilder of the Mayo Clinic, who coined the term in the 1960s. Advancements in research during this decade revealed that medium-chain triglycerides (MCTs) produced even more ketones per unit of energy. Consequently, the ketogenic diet prescribed to epileptic patients was revised by Peter Huttenlocher, which integrated MCT oil to constitute 60% of the sufferer's daily caloric intake. This meant that a wider assortment of meals were now available to patients. From this was born the ketogenic diet as we know it today.

KETOSIS
Nature's Balance

The basic principle of the ketogenic diet is that it is a low-carbohydrate, high-fat diet. Specifically, you want to keep your carb consumption between 5% to 10% of your daily intake, fat between 60% to 75%, and protein between 15% to 30%. This particular proportion of nutrients will allow your body to produce ketones as an energy source, which is what occurs when your body enters into a state known as ketosis.

With an average balanced diet, carbohydrates are processed by being turned into glucose for energy. When ketosis is achieved, conversely, your body begins to use ketones, which are produced during the transfer of fat to energy. By maintaining ketosis you transition into a metabolic state in which your body burns these ketones. Ketosis happens naturally when your glucose levels are low. As we've already seen, it can be used to mitigate symptoms of epilepsy and can also be instrumental to weight loss, which can of course help boost your self-esteem and overall well-being. Not only that but ketosis can help strengthen your body's resistance to insulin, meaning it is an effective treatment for diabetics. Let's go back to ketones for a moment. Ketones or ketone bodies are byproducts of the breakdown of fat into energy. Their production works like this:

- When there isn't enough glucose in your body, your glycogen levels drop and eventually get depleted.
- Your body now has to find alternative resources to fuel itself – namely fat
- This is where ketones come in. They are produced by the liver to fuel your body.
- When you have reached this state, you are said to be under ketosis.

Let's remind ourselves of the three ketone bodies that arise from this process:

- acetoacetate
- acetone
- β-hydroxybutyrate

Carbohydrates are an obvious, and often delicious, source of energy. Simple sugars from foods like bread, rice and candy are broken down quickly and easily, and will provide you will enough fuel to get through the day. A steady carb intake from breakfast to supper allows your body to function smoothly. But here's where we run into a problem: any excess simple sugars will be stored as fat to be burned later; for example, if you skip a meal. If you are consistently consuming more than your body needs to survive, this will most likely lead to weight gain. A fat store is of course necessary in order to keep you going between meals, but in today's world of sedentary workdays and XL portion sizes, many of us keep a continuous store of fat that we will never burn, and consequently gain a significant amount of weight.

At times when you do not have a steady source of carbohydrates, your body has to draw fat from its stores to be burned for energy. The burning of fat is called ketosis, and the byproducts of this process are ketones. In this way we can regard ketosis as the body's natural 'back-up plan', an alternative to burning carbohydrates, in the interest of survival. As you might expect, ketosis is an excellent means of losing weight as it means you are now burning fat instead of the carbohydrates entering your system. Unfortunately, entering ketosis takes time, and any progress you have made towards reaching this state is instantly negated as soon as you go back to eating carbohydrate-based foods, as your body reverts to burning sugars. Luckily you can substitute carbs with proteins and fats, in order to push your body into a state of ketosis.

The maximum amount of carbs you can consume daily on a keto diet will of course vary from person to person. However, the threshold generally sits at 50-60 grams per day, roughly 10-15 grams per meal, before exiting ketosis. 15 grams is equal to one small piece of fruit. Such a low amount of carbs must be obtained from healthy choices, in particular from vegetables. A basic ketogenic meal combines proteins from meat or fish with a large helping of non-starchy vegetables, like salad, zucchini, or asparagus. Since your fat intake is largely unrestricted, healthy fats like olive oil and avocado can be used to compensate for the carbohydrate-rich starches that will now be missing from your diet, like rice and potatoes.

Maintaining ketosis is the key to forcing your body into a metabolic state. Starvation is not the objective here, but rather carbohydrate starvation. Your body's innate ability to adapt to drastic changes in diet means that when you load it with fats instead of carbs, you will start to burn ketones as an energy source rather than sugars. Eventually, you will burn ketones at such a rate that you'll see the weight dropping off.

Ketoacidosis

It must be underlined that ketosis is different from ketoacidosis, which is a metabolic state to which sufferers of type 1 diabetes are particularly susceptible. Ketoacidosis occurs when there are dangerously high levels of ketones in the bloodstream (between three and five times higher than those you get with ketosis). Ketosis and ketoacidosis are sometimes confused; the important distinction to make is that while ketoacidosis can be life-threatening, ketosis is a natural process of the body that, when properly monitored, has numerous health benefits.

Ketosis Achieved

Ketosis is a form of acidosis (a high saturation of acid in body tissues or fluids). The presence of ketones in your blood means that the pH balance of your body is decreased. Ketone bodies can be utilized by the heart, muscle tissue, and the kidneys, for energy production, and can also provide a source of energy to the brain. Crucially, ketosis is an extremely effective way of breaking down fat. Reaching ketosis might seem like a daunting task to newcomers to the diet but fear not. On the whole, it is pretty straightforward, provided you follow some basic guidelines.

•   Limit carbs – Remember that you need to be focusing on limiting your total carb intake as well as your net carb intake. Ideally, you should keep your net carbs below 20g a day, and your total carbs below 35g.

- Limit protein consumption – Many folks coming from other diets might forget to limit their protein intake in tandem with their carb intake. Too much protein can diminish your ketone levels and therefore restrict your ability to enter ketosis. If you want to achieve that coveted lean body type, you want to eat about 0.6-0.8 grams of protein per pound consumed.
- Don't fuss over fat – Though it might seem counterintuitive to weight loss, fat intake is a priority with the keto diet, as it becomes your primary source of energy. Contrary to popular belief, starving yourself is not conducive to effective and sustainable weight loss, so avoid this at all costs.
- Drink water – When taking on the keto diet, make it your goal to drink a gallon of water a day. Though this might sound like a lot, staying hydrated is crucial to ensuring your body functions as normal and to managing your levels of hunger.
- Cut the snacks – Random spikes in insulin levels throughout the day can greatly impede your ability to lose weight, so avoid snacking if you want to maintain your progress.
- Fast – Fasting is a great way to raise your ketone levels. A good habit to get into is simply skipping certain meals. Which meal you skip is up to you. Designate an 'eating window' of between four and seven hours and leave the remaining time for fasting. You might consider engaging in extended fasting periods every once in a while, – cleanses of between 24 and 28 hours during which you do not eat at all.
- Exercise – There's no question that exercise is beneficial to everyone. To get the most out of your keto diet, increase your current daily exercise routine by 20 or 30 minutes, even if it's just a leisurely walk. Every little helps towards regulating your blood sugar and promoting weight loss.
- Consider taking supplements – While this is not a necessity, supplements have nutritional benefits that can nicely complement your keto diet.

Foods to Avoid

Committing to the keto diet requires a certain amount of discipline with regards to your eating habits. To optimize your chances of success, there are some foods you should avoid at all costs. These include:

- Grains, in all forms. This means no rice, corn, oats, wheat, barley, pasta, bread, cookies, crackers, and so forth.
- Factory-farmed fish and pork. Organic and local is always better quality.
- Processed foods, which are often high in sugar.
- Artificial sweeteners.
- Refined fats and oils, such as canola oil and soybean oil.
- Foods that claim to be "low-carb" or "zero-carb" – these labels are often deceptive.
- Milk, as it is quite high in carbs.
- Alcoholic and sweet beverages.
- Soy products, as many of them are highly processed and they can mess with your hormone levels.

KETO SIDE EFFECTS
The Worthwhile Struggle

You may feel overwhelmed by the surplus of resources that are out there, many of which give conflicting advice as to how to achieve optimal ketosis. For me, there is no shortcut – the only way to figure out how best to reach ketosis is to jump straight in and make the appropriate changes to your diet. You might like to try measuring your ketone levels with urine strip tests, but this method is sometimes inaccurate and not easy on the pocket. A cheaper and more useful alternative is to learn to recognize the physical signs that you are entering a state of ketosis:

• More urination – Ketones can induce a diuretic response. The keto diet increases the volume of acetoacetate in your body, which is excreted in the urine. As a result, you might find yourself making trips to the bathroom more often than normal.

• Thirst and dry mouth – You can attribute these side effects to the increased urination. To fight these symptoms, it's extra important to drink lots of water, so as to replenish your electrolytes.

• Bad breath – Acetone, one of our three ketone bodies, is excreted into the mouth during ketosis. Some people find this makes their breath smell like ripe fruit, while other describe the smell as more akin to nail polish remover. Thankfully, this will go away with time.

• Reduced hunger and increased energy – Once you're past the keto flu, you will find your energy is higher, your state of mind clearer, and your hunger reduced.

• Keto Flu – A common phenomenon experienced by many newcomers to the diet, the 'keto flu' may manifest as mild cramps, nausea, headaches and fatigue. Fortunately, it is temporary, lasting just a few days. Despite the name, the keto flu (also known as the 'low-carb flu') is not actually a kind of influenza. It is so-called because many newcomers to the keto diet experience a number of flu-like symptoms in the early stages of their keto transformation.

There are two main reasons why the keto flu occurs:

1 Urination – More frequent trips to the bathroom: Increased urination leads to a considerable loss of electrolytes and water. You can preemptively combat this problem by drinking a bouillon cube dissolved in water.

2 Withdrawal – Remember, your body is going through a major transition! It now has to adjust to a significant drop in carb intake and create new enzymes in order to process increased amounts of fat. This is hard work for your body, and you may feel lethargic as a result. To ease this, you should try decreasing your carb intake gradually, rather than quitting cold turkey.

Increasing your water consumption and replacing lost electrolytes will effectively combat or even eradicate the keto flu. At the beginning of your transition you should try to eat less than 15 grams of carbohydrates a day, then increase this number little by little over time. Nothing worth doing is easy, but thankfully the drawbacks of the keto diet are few and, for the most part, easily alleviated. Here are some other notable side effects of the ketogenic diet, and suggestions as to how you can deal with them.

- Fatigue and irritability – High ketone levels can positively impact your physical wellbeing in a number of ways, but they are also linked to increased tiredness and quicker exertion during exercise. Make sure you are getting enough sleep during the early days of your transition and avoid particularly strenuous exercise if necessary.
- 'Brain fog' – Your altered metabolism and hormonal state may cause decreased mental clarity or 'brain fog.' This is a common side effect of total carbohydrate withdrawal, which is why you should avoid going cold turkey and instead decrease your carbohydrate intake gradually and steadily.
- Change in lipids – An important tenet of the ketogenic diet is not only to up your fat intake but also to watch what kinds of fats you are consuming. Saturated fats are known to increase cholesterol levels, so make sure they do not outbalance the non-saturated fats in your diet.
- Micronutrient deficiencies – Low-carb foods are often lacking in important nutrients like magnesium, potassium and iron. Taking supplements is an excellent way of compensating for this.
- Ketoacidosis – If your diet is poorly-planned, you may be at risk of developing ketoacidosis, which is characterized by extremely high ketone levels. This is especially harmful to sufferers of diabetes, so make sure you organize your diet so as to keep your ketone levels within a healthy range. Additionally, it is important to know how to recognize the signs.

KETO BENEFITS

Diets are often met with criticism, and the keto diet is not immune to controversy. In particular, some have raised concerns about the high fat intake that keto requires, as fatty foods are known to raise cholesterol and cause heart disease. However, studies have shown that when carefully planned and adhered to, low-carb regimens win out against all others. They are not only advantageous to those trying to lose weight but come with a whole host of extra health benefits that will improve your overall well-being. In some cases, the keto diet can even reduce your cholesterol levels. Let's delve deeper into the various perks of the keto diet. The main process at play with the ketogenic diet is ketosis. Entering this metabolic state has been shown to positively impact the body in a number of ways, even if you are only on the diet for a brief period of time. Ketosis itself has a number of benefits. It has been shown to:

- improves the body's ability to draw on fats as an energy source.
- spare your proteins, as your body starts to use ketones as fuel instead.
- lower insulin levels in the body, which influences the secretion of growth hormones.

Now let's get to grips with some of the overall benefits of the ketogenic diet.

- Suppressed appetite – Most diets require you to reduce your overall food consumption, and the consequential hunger is likely to cause you some discomfort. Hunger is a stumbling block for many, and a notable reason why so many dieters fail. Low-carb diets, on the other hand, have the added benefit of reducing your appetite. Cutting carbs and substituting them with fats and proteins means you cut your caloric intake without going hungry.

- Increased potential for weight loss – Compared with many other popular diets, low-carb regimens promote a much faster rate of weight loss. Low levels of carbohydrates help reduce the excess water in the body, which often accounts for a considerable percentage of our unwanted pounds. Moreover, the keto diet diminishes insulin levels, flushing the body of the surplus sodium that retains the extra weight.

- Reduction of triglycerides – The presence of triglycerides, or fat molecules, in the body correlates strongly with illnesses like heart disease. The fewer carbs you consume, the fewer triglycerides there are in your system, which is great news for your long-term health.

- More good cholesterol – You may be under the impression that cholesterol is universally bad for you, but there is, in fact, a form of cholesterol that actually reduces the risk of heart disease: high-density lipoprotein or HDL. The increased consumption of fats associated with the keto diet raises levels of HDL. HDL is not only a positive addition to your system, but it helps eradicate bad cholesterol (LDL) from your bloodstream.

- Reduced blood sugar and insulin levels – Carbohydrate-rich foods are broken down into simple sugars by our digestive system, which inevitably elevates blood sugar levels. Insulin is needed to combat these toxins. A high-carb diet, maintained over a long period of time, can interfere with the body's ability to produce insulin, leading to type 2 diabetes. The ketogenic diet is advantageous in this regard, as it lowers blood sugar and insulin levels significantly.

- Natural treatment for cancer – According to some researchers, disciplined regulation of your body's metabolic functions can potentially reduce the risk of and even treat cancer. Low-carb diets deprive cancerous cells of fuel, as these types of cells feed off of glucose and cannot adapt to the shift in energy sources involved with ketosis. As a result, the keto diet may be able to prevent cancerous cells from spreading.

- Treatment for metabolic syndrome – Metabolic syndrome is a serious medical condition which increases the risk of heart disease, diabetes, and stroke. There are numerous symptoms, including:
  - Low levels of HDL
  - High triglyceride levels
  - Raised fasting blood sugar levels
  - Elevated blood pressure
- Therapy for some brain disorders – Certain parts of our brains rely exclusively on glucose for fuel. This is why our livers need to derive glucose from protein if our carb intake is low. However, larger sections of the brain are capable of using ketones for fuel. With the keto diet, certain biochemical changes may occur in the brain which can potentially eradicate the circuit system that is responsible for seizures. Think back to Hugh Conklin and his use of the ketogenic diet as treatment for sufferers of epileptic seizures – 50% of his patients reported their condition was greatly improved.

KETO FATS

Good Fats

Fats are integral to the keto diet. In addition to consuming high proportions of fats, it is vital that you make sure you are consuming the right varieties. Let's cut through all the confusion surrounding the good and bad kinds of fat and discuss which fats you should be aiming to integrate into your ketogenic diet.

We divide the 'good fats' into four distinct categories:

- Saturated fats
- Monounsaturated fatty acids (MUFAs)
- Polyunsaturated fatty acids (PUFAs)
- Trans fats (naturally occurring)

All fats constitute a combination of the above varieties but are named according to the kind that is most dominant in their makeup. We will now take a look at each type of fat and consider which ones you should be including as part of your ketogenic diet. This way, you will be able to make quick and informed decisions as to how best to fuel your mind and body.

Saturated Fats

Saturated fats get a bad rep – many of us have been advised to avoid them because of the potential harmful effects they can have on our heart health. However, recent research has shown that there is no strong correlation between saturated fats and heart disease. After all, saturated fats have been a major component of the human diet for millennia. There are in fact numerous ways in which saturated fats can be advantageous to us.

Some foods with saturated fats in them contain medium-chain triglycerides (MCTs), particularly coconut oil, butter and palm oil. MCTs are easily digestible and are converted to energy in the liver. As a result, they are highly beneficial to those who want to lose weight or improve their performance during physical activity.

Here are some further benefits:

- Boosted immune system.
- Improved HDL-to-LDL cholesterol ratio.
- Improved bone density.
- Increased levels of HDL cholesterol to remove LDL from the arteries.
- Increased production of important hormones like cortisol and testosterone.

Foods which are rich in saturated fats include:

- Butter
- Cocoa butter
- Coconut oil
- Cream
- Eggs
- Lard
- Palm oil

- Red meat

Monounsaturated Fats

Monounsaturated fatty acids (MUFAs) differ from saturated fats in that they are pretty much universally embraced as a 'good' kind of fat. Numerous studies have revealed a link between MUFAs and certain positive outcomes like insulin resistance and good cholesterol. Other health benefits include:

- Lower blood pressure
- Decreased risk of developing heart disease
- Decrease in belly fat

The best sources of MUFAs are:

- Avocados and avocado oil
- Extra virgin olive oil
- Lard and bacon fat
- Macadamia nut oil

Polyunsaturated Fats

How you prepare foods containing polyunsaturated fatty acids (PUFAs) is critical. When PUFAs are subjected to heat, they can create free radicals (uncharged molecules) which cause inflammation and have even been linked to cancer and heart disease. This means that for the most part PUFAs should be eaten cold, and never cooked.

You can get PUFAs from processed oils and other heart-friendly sources. The right kinds of PUFAs have immense health benefits when adopted into a balanced diet. Some such fats are Omega 3 and Omega 6, which are the primary components of many superfoods such as salmon and flaxseed.

Integrating PUFAs into your diet is therefore crucial. An ideal ratio of Omega 3 to Omega 6 stands at around 1:1 – however, most Westerners consume a ratio of 1:30! A good balance between Omega 3 and Omega 6 greatly decreases the risk of developing the following:

- Autoimmune disorders and other inflammatory diseases
- Heart disease
- Stroke
- Depression and ADHD

PUFA-rich foods include:

- Avocado oil
- Chia seeds
- Extra virgin olive oil
- Flaxseeds and flaxseed oil
- Sesame oil
- Walnuts

Trans Fats

You might double-take at seeing trans fats listed as 'good' fats, but they do in fact have a right to be termed as such. Though most trans fats are indeed unhealthy, one particular naturally occurring variety is decidedly beneficial: vaccenic acid. Vaccenic acid can be absorbed from grass-fed meats and dairy products.

The potential health benefits of this type of trans fat include:

- Lower risk of developing diabetes and obesity
- Lower risk of developing heart disease
- Protection against cancer

The best sources of healthy and natural trans fats are:

- Butter
- Yogurt
- Grass-fed animal products

Bad Fats

Many people are drawn to the keto diet because it permits you to eat foods that, being high in fat, are satisfying and delicious. However, the idea that keto dieters can consume all the fat they want is a common misconception. On the contrary, there are several 'bad fats' which you should take the utmost care to avoid if you wish to achieve the best possible results. Remember, the quality of the food you eat should always be a number-one priority.

You may be familiar with these kinds of fats, as they are present in many of the sweet and snack foods many of us enjoy. You may also already know that they are extremely damaging to your physical well-being. Artificial trans fats are the product of the processing of polyunsaturated fats. For this reason, you must try to consume only unprocessed PUFAs that have not been heated or modified in any way.

Trans fats are particularly harmful as they may lead to:

- An increased risk of cancer
- An increased risk of heart disease
- Inflammatory health issues
- A decrease in HDL cholesterol and an increase of LDL cholesterol

Here are some common sources of trans fats which you should aim to cut from your diet:

- Hydrogenated and partially hydrogenated oils that are in processed products like cookies, crackers, margarine, and fast food.
- Processed vegetable oils like cottonseed, sunflower, safflower, soybean, and canola oil.

Conclusion

Saturated fats are not the boogeymen they've often been portrayed to be, but the best fats are those which are unprocessed. Processed and packaged foods are major stoppers to weight loss and heart health, so avoid them at all costs. At the end of the day, the main objective of the keto diet is to improve your overall well-being. This involves not only maintaining a good macro ratio but selecting the right kinds of foods for your health and physical condition.

KETO SUCCESS
Staying Focused

The keto diet doesn't come without its stumbling blocks, so here are some essential tips for staying on track as you progress further down the Instant Pot road.

- Practice intermittent fasting – Before jumping straight in, steadily reduce your carb intake in the days leading up to your fast days. Fast days should be divided into two phases:
- Building phase – The period of time between your first and last meal.
- Cleaning phase – The period of time between your last and first meal. To start, try a cleaning phase of between 12 and 16 hours and a building phase of between 8 and 12 hours. As your body adjusts to the change, you will find yourself in a position to tackle a 4-6-hour building time and an 18-20-hour cleaning phase.
- Consume salt – Too much sodium is generally deemed as unhealthy. However, a low-carb diet necessitates a high salt intake, as this type of regimen reduces your insulin levels and flushes out higher amounts of sodium from your kidneys. As a result, your sodium/potassium ratio is disrupted. Here are some tips to counteract this change:
- Exercise regularly – Daily rigorous exercise can help activate glucose molecules called GLUT-4 which are needed to return glucose to fat and muscle tissues. Additionally, it can double the amount of protein present in both the liver and the muscles.
- Work on improving bowel movements – Many keto dieters experience constipation. Thankfully, this can be easily combatted by consuming fermented foods like sauerkraut, coconut water, and kimchi. You may also want to try supplements like magnesium. Green tea, too, has been shown to add to the levels of calcium, magnesium and potassium in your body, all of which are useful in fighting constipation.
- Watch how much protein you eat – Protein is integral to the keto diet but maintaining a proper balance is a must. If you eat too many protein-rich foods, you will end up converting the amino acids into glucose (through a process called gluconeogenesis). In the initial stages of your keto diet, vary the amounts of protein you consume in order to get a feel of how much is too much.
- Pick your carbs wisely – The few carb-rich foods you do consume should be selected very carefully. It is best to stick to starchy veggies and fruits like berries, apples, lemons, and oranges. For a quick morning hit, blend them into a healthy green smoothie.
- Take MCT oil – High-quality MCTs are extremely effective in replenishing the energy levels you deplete through the day. MCT oil can be used for cooking, as well as added to beverages like coffee, tea, smoothies, protein shakes, and so on.
- Minimize your stress – Stress is a major factor in decreased energy levels, so constant stress may serve as a threat to your keto success. If you find yourself especially prone to stress at the moment, it may be wise to avoid dieting until you're in a better position to deal with the blow to your energy levels.

- Improve the quality of your sleep – Sleep is essential for managing stress, among other things. Make sure your bedroom is conducive to a good night's rest. This means sleeping in a comfortable bed, in a darkened room no warmer than 70 degrees. Most adults function best on 7 to 9 hours of sleep every night, though a particularly stressful lifestyle may require even longer.
- Eat ghee – Ghee works well as a butter substitute, as it can be used in more or less all the same ways and is exponentially healthier. Try frying meat or vegetables in it for a high-fat, healthy meal.
- Seek out Omega 3s – If you find it hard to integrate Omega-3-rich foods into your diet, then you might consider taking supplements. You should make sure your Omega 3 intake matches your Omega 6s. Omega 3 is an extremely beneficial kind of fat, which is crucial to the keto diet.
- Avoid alcohol – It may be hard to kiss the booze goodbye, but it is well-attested that alcohol impedes weight loss. Stay focused on your goals and order a glass of tonic water at the bar instead.
- Drink lemon water – Lemon water is a tasty and refreshing alternative to tap water that has the added benefit of balancing your pH levels.
- Avoid 'sugar-free' products – These labels may sound appealing, but the vast majority of products advertised as 'sugar-free' or 'light' contain more carbs than the original!
- Say goodbye to low-fat products – Anything low in fat is not suitable for the keto diet. Maintaining high percentages of fat in your diet is essential – otherwise the protein you eat will be converted to sugars.
- Buy a food scale – Food scales are a great utensil to keep handy in your kitchen as they help you to accurately monitor what you are putting into your body. They are indispensable in tracking your carb and overall caloric intake. Invest in your success – get a high-quality, durable scale with a conversion button, automatic shutdown, tare function, and a removable plate.
- Stay carb-savvy – To tackle the inevitable carb cravings, it is a good idea to make yourself aware of the many alternatives that exist.
- Shirataki noodles – are made from yams and make a great low-carb alternative to pasta.
- Cauliflower rice – basically, shredded cauliflower, mimics the texture and neutral taste of white or brown rice.
- Spaghetti squash – can be cut into the shape of noodles with the aid of a spiralizer or a fork. It tastes great and amounts to less than half the carbs and calories of conventional noodles.
- Heavy whipping cream or almond milk – go great in your coffee instead of regular creamer, which is rich in calories.
- Low-carb bread and tortillas – are available for those who just can't seem to kick the bread addiction.
- Protein powder – can satisfy your sweet tooth in a shake or smoothie. It comes in a wide variety of flavors and is easily incorporated into practically any meal. Plus, needless to say, its high protein content is an added benefit, offering an easy boost to your keto diet

30 DAY MEAL PLAN
Week 1

- Each day will be between 1,500-1,700 calories (designed for weight loss).
- This meal plan is designed for 1 person. If you would like to use them for multiple people, simply multiply the ingredient quantities by the total number of people.
- Be flexible! Feel free to replace any of the recipes or ingredients with your personal choices and adjust the ingredient amounts to fit your macros and situation.
- If you follow a very strict keto diet, make sure to personalize this meal plan (including the snack list suggestion at the end) to make it work for you.

Monday	*Cristy's Pancakes 1*	*Monkey Salad 1*	*Grilled Ham & Cheese 1*
Tuesday	*Breakfast Tea 1*	*Jarlsberg Lunch Omelet 1*	*Prosciutto Spinach Salad 1*
Wednesday	*Sausage Quiche 1*	*Mu Shu Lunch Pork 1*	*Cabbage & Beef Casserole 1*
Thursday	*Breakfast Sausage Casserole 1*	*Fiery Jalapeno Poppers 1*	*Easy Zoodles & Turkey Balls 1*
Friday	*Scrambled Mug Eggs 1*	Bacon & Chicken Patties 1	Lasagna Spaghetti Squash 1
Saturday	*Banana Chia Seed Pudding 1*	*Cauliflower Rice Chicken Curry 1*	*Blue Cheese Chicken Wedges 1*
Sunday	*Strawberry Rhubarb Parfait 1*	*'I Love Bacon' 1*	*'Oh so good' Salad 1*

Week 2

Monday	*Cristy's Pancakes 1*	*Duck Fat Ribeye 1*	*Stuffed Chicken Rolls 1*
Tuesday	*Strawberry Rhubarb Parfait 1*	*Jarlsberg Lunch Omelet 1*	*Chicken in a Blanket 1*
Wednesday	*Sausage Egg Muffins 1*	*Dijon Halibut Steak 1*	*Riced Cauliflower & Curry Chicken 1*
Thursday	*Breakfast Sausage Casserole 1*	*Roast Beef Lettuce Wraps 1*	*Mashed Garlic Turnips 1*
Friday	*Salmon Omelet 1*	*Bacon & Chicken Patties 1*	*Chicken Tenders 1*
Saturday	*Banana Chia Seed Pudding 1*	*Cheddar Bacon Burst 1*	*Fat Bombs 1*
Sunday	*Spinach Eggs and Cheese 1*	*Meatballs 1*	*Nearly Pizza1*

Week 3

Monday	*Cristy's Pancakes 1*	*Lemon Dill Trout 1*	*Gluten Free Gratin 1*
Tuesday	*Bangin' Casserole 1*	*Jarlsberg Lunch Omelet 1*	*Prosciutto Spinach Salad 1*
Wednesday	*Sausage Egg Muffins 1*	*Easy Slider 1*	*Sausage Balls 1*
Thursday	*Bacon Cups 1*	*'I Love Bacon' 1*	*Turkey Avocado Rolls 1*
Friday	*Scotch Eggs 1*	*Cast-Iron Cheesy Chicken 1*	*Lasagna Spaghetti Squash 1*
Saturday	*Fried Eggs 1*	*Bacon Chops 1*	*Bacon Scallops 1*
Sunday	*Hash Browns 1*	*'No Potato' Shepherd's Pie 1*	*Buffalo Chicken Salad 1*

Week 4

Monday	_Breakfast Cheesy Sausage_	_Cheesy Bacon Butternut Squash_	_Browned Butter Asparagus_
Tuesday	_Cauliflower Toast with Avocado_	_Jalapeño Popper Stuffed Zucchini_	_Roasted Brussels Sprouts_
Wednesday	_Keto Avocado Toast_	_Turkey Carrot Roll Up_	_Mexican Taco Casserole_
Thursday	_Chocolate Chip Waffles_	_Sweet & Savory Chicken_	_Hamburger Patties_
Friday	_Egg Crepes with Avocados_	_Lemon Pepper Green Beans_	_Keto Dinner Mussels_
Saturday	_Ham & Cheese Pockets_	_Cumin Spiced Beef Wraps_	_Thai Curry Insta Pork_
Sunday	_Clementine & Pistachio_	_Mahi Mahi Stew_	_Mediterranean Turkey Cutlets_

BREAKFASTS
Pancakes

Prep + Cook Time: 15 minutes | Servings: 2

Amount per **one** serving: 260 cal., 23g fat, 7g protein & 3g carbs.

INGREDIENTS

- 2 tbsp coconut oil
- 1 tsp maple extract
- 2 tbsp cashew milk
- 2 eggs

INSTRUCTIONS

1.   Add the oil to a skillet. Add a quarter-cup of the batter and fry until golden on each side. Continue adding the remaining batter.

Breakfast Sandwich

Prep + Cook Time: 10 minutes | Servings: 2

Amount per **one** serving: 600 cal., 50g fat, 12g protein & 7g carbs.

INGREDIENTS

- 2 oz/60g cheddar cheese
- 1/6 oz/30g smoked ham
- 2 tbsp butter
- 4 eggs

INSTRUCTIONS

1.   Fry all the eggs and sprinkle the pepper and salt on them.
2.   Place an egg down as the sandwich base. Top with the ham and cheese and a drop or two of Tabasco.
3.   Place the other egg on top and enjoy.

Egg Muffins

Prep + Cook Time: 30 minutes | Servings: 6

Amount per **one** serving: 190 cal., 15g fat, 7g protein & 4g carbs.

INGREDIENTS

- 1 tbsp green pesto
- 3 oz/75g shredded cheese
- 5 oz/150g cooked bacon
- 1 scallion, chopped
- 6 eggs

INSTRUCTIONS

1. You should set your oven to 350°F/175°C.
2. Place liners in a regular cupcake tin. This will help with easy removal and storage.
3. Beat the eggs with pepper, salt, and the pesto. Mix in the cheese.
4. Pour the eggs into the cupcake tin and top with the bacon and scallion.
5. Cook for 15-20 minutes, or until the egg is set.

Bacon & Eggs

Prep + Cook Time: 5 minutes | Servings: 4

Amount per **one** serving: 80 cal., 7g fat, 14g protein & 2g carbs.

INGREDIENTS

- Parsley
- Cherry tomatoes
- 5 1/3 oz/150g bacon
- 8 eggs

INSTRUCTIONS

1. Fry up the bacon and put it to the side.
2. Scramble the eggs in the bacon grease, with some pepper and salt. If you want, scramble in some cherry tomatoes. Sprinkle with some parsley and enjoy.

Eggs on the Go

Prep + Cook Time: 10 minutes | Servings: 12
Amount per **one** serving: 75 cal., 6g fat, 8g protein & 1g carbs.

INGREDIENTS
- 4 oz/110g bacon, cooked
- Pepper
- Salt
- 12 eggs

INSTRUCTIONS
1. You should set your oven to 400°F/200°C.
2. Place liners in a regular cupcake tin. This will help with easy removal and storage.
3. Crack an egg into each of the cups and sprinkle some bacon onto each of them. Season with some pepper and salt.
4. Bake for 15 minutes, or until the eggs are set.

Cream Cheese Pancakes

Prep + Cook Time: 10 minutes | Servings: 1
Amount per **one** serving: 340 cal., 30g fat, 7g protein & 3g carbs.

INGREDIENTS
- 2 oz cream cheese
- 2 eggs
- ½ tsp cinnamon
- 1 tbsp keto coconut flour
- ½ to 1 packet of Stevia

INSTRUCTIONS
1. Mix together all the ingredients until smooth.
2. Heat up a non-stick pan or skillet with butter or coconut oil on medium-high.
3. Make them as you would normal pancakes.
4. Cook it on one side and then flip to cook the other side!
5. Top with some butter and/or sugar-free syrup.

Breakfast Mix

Prep + Cook Time: 15 minutes | Servings: 1

Amount per **one** serving: 150 cal., 9g fat, 8g protein & 4g carbs.

INGREDIENTS

- 5 tbsp coconut flakes, unsweetened
- 7 tbsp hemp seeds
- 5 tbsp flaxseed, ground
- 2 tbsp sesame, ground
- 2 tbsp cocoa, dark, unsweetened

INSTRUCTIONS

1. Grind the flaxseed and the sesame.
2. Make sure you only grind the sesame seeds for a very short period.
3. Mix all ingredients in a jar and shake it well.
4. Keep refrigerated until ready to eat.
5. Serve softened with black coffee or even with still water and add coconut oil if you want to increase the fat content. It also blends well with cream or with mascarpone cheese.

Breakfast Muffins

Prep + Cook Time: 30 minutes | Servings: 1

Amount per **one** serving: 150 cal.,11g fat, 7g protein & 2g carbs.

INGREDIENTS

- 1 medium egg
- ¼ cup heavy cream
- 1 slice cooked bacon (cured, pan-fried, cooked)
- 1 oz cheddar cheese
- Salt and black pepper (to taste)

INSTRUCTIONS

1. Preheat your oven to 350°F/175°C.
2. In a bowl, mix the eggs with the cream, salt and pepper.
3. Spread into muffin tins and fill the cups half full.
4. Place 1 slice of bacon into each muffin hole and half ounce of cheese on top of each muffin.
5. Bake for around 15-20 minutes or until slightly browned.
6. Add another ½ oz of cheese onto each muffin and broil until the cheese is slightly browned. Serve!

Egg Porridge

Prep + Cook Time: 15 minutes | Servings: 2

Amount per **one** serving: 604 cal., 45g fat, 8g protein & 2.8g carbs.

INGREDIENTS

- 2 organic free-range eggs
- 1/3 cup organic heavy cream without food additives
- 2 packages of your preferred sweetener
- 2 tbsp grass-fed butter ground organic cinnamon to taste

INSTRUCTIONS

1. In a bowl add the eggs, cream and sweetener, and mix together.
2. Melt the butter in a saucepan over a medium heat. Lower the heat once the butter is melted.
3. Combine together with the egg and cream mixture.
4. While Cooking, mix until it thickens and curdles.
5. When you see the first signs of curdling, remove the saucepan immediately from the heat.
6. Pour the porridge into a bowl. Sprinkle cinnamon on top and serve immediately.

Eggs Florentine

Prep + Cook Time: 20 minutes | Servings: 2

Amount per **one** serving: 180 cal., 10g fat, 7g protein & 5g carbs.

INGREDIENTS

- 1 cup washed, fresh spinach leaves
- 2 tbsp freshly grated parmesan cheese
- Sea salt and pepper
- 1 tbsp white vinegar
- 2 eggs

INSTRUCTIONS

1. Cook the spinach the microwave or steam until wilted.
2. Sprinkle with parmesan cheese and seasoning.
3. Slice into bite-size pieces and place on a plate.
4. Simmer a pan of water and add the vinegar. Stir quickly with a spoon.
5. Break an egg into the center. Turn off the heat and cover until set.
6. Repeat with the second egg.
7. Place the eggs on top of the spinach and serve.

Spanish Omelet

Prep + Cook Time: 15 minutes | Servings: 3

Amount per **one** serving: 160 cal., 15g fat, 7g protein & 4g carbs.

INGREDIENTS

- 3 eggs
- Cayenne or black pepper
- ½ cup finely chopped vegetables of your choosing.

INSTRUCTIONS

1.   In a pan on high heat, stir-fry the vegetables in extra virgin olive oil until lightly crispy.
2.   Cook the eggs with one tablespoon of water and a pinch of pepper.
3.   When almost cooked, top with the vegetables and flip to cook briefly.
4.   Serve

Cristy's Pancakes

Prep + Cook Time: 10 minutes | Servings: 1

Amount per **one** serving: 300 cal., 30g fat, 8g protein & 2 carbs.

INGREDIENTS

- 1 scoop of KetogenX Vanilla
- 1 tbsp almond or hazelnut meal
- 2 tbsp water
- 1 egg

INSTRUCTIONS

1.   Add the ingredients together in a bowl and mix together.
2.   Pour the mixture into a frying pan, cook on a medium heat for approximately 2 to 3 minutes on each side. (Watch carefully as it may burn quickly.)
3.   Serve buttered with a handful of mixed berries.

Breakfast Tea

Prep + Cook Time: 5 minutes | Servings: 1

Amount per **one** serving: 110 cal., 12g fat, 1g protein & 1g carbs.

INGREDIENTS

- 16 oz water
- 2 tea bags
- 1 tbsp ghee
- 1 tbsp coconut oil
- ½ tsp vanilla extract

INSTRUCTIONS

1. Make the tea and put it to one aside.
2. In a bowl, melt the ghee.
3. Add the coconut oil and vanilla to the melted ghee.
4. Pour the tea from a cup into a Nutribullet cup.
5. Screw on the lid and blend thoroughly.

Sausage Quiche

Prep + Cook Time: 35 minutes | Servings: 6

Amount per **one** serving: 335 cal., 30g fat, 11g protein & 2g carbs.

INGREDIENTS

- 12 large eggs
- 1 cup heavy cream
- 1 tsp black pepper
- 12 oz sugar-free breakfast sausage
- 2 cups shredded cheddar cheese

INSTRUCTIONS

1. Preheat your oven to 375°F/190°C.
2. In a large bowl, whisk the eggs, heavy cream, sausage and pepper together.
3. Add the breakfast sausage and cheddar cheese.
4. Pour the mixture into a greased casserole dish.
5. Bake for 25 minutes.
6. Cut into 12 squares and serve hot.

Breakfast Sausage Casserole

Prep + Cook Time: 50 minutes | Servings: 4

Amount per **one** serving: 290 cal., 25g fat, 12g protein & 1g carbs.

INGREDIENTS

- 8 eggs, beaten
- 1 head chopped cauliflower
- 1 lb sausage, cooked and crumbled
- 2 cups heavy whipping cream
- 1 cup sharp cheddar cheese, grated

INSTRUCTIONS

1. Cook the sausage as usual.
2. In a large bowl, mix the sausage, heavy whipping cream, chopped cauliflower, cheese and eggs.
3. Pour into a greased casserole dish.
4. Cook for 45 minutes at 350°F/175°C, or until firm.
5. Top with cheese and serve.

Scrambled Mug Eggs

Prep + Cook Time: 5 minutes | Servings: 1

Amount per **one** serving: 330 cal., 30g fat, 12g protein & 1g carbs.

INGREDIENTS

- 1 mug
- 2 eggs
- Salt and pepper
- Shredded cheese
- Your favorite buffalo wing sauce

INSTRUCTIONS

1. Crack the eggs into a mug and whisk until blended.
2. Put the mug into your microwave and cook for 1.5 – 2 minutes, depending on the power of your microwave.
3. Leave for a few minutes and remove from the microwave.
4. Sprinkle with salt and pepper. Add your desired amount of cheese on top.
5. Using a fork, mix everything together.
6. Then add your favorite buffalo or hot sauce and mix again.
7. Serve!

Banana Chia Seed Pudding

Prep + Cook Time: 1-2 days | Servings: 1

Amount per **one** serving: 130 cal., 12g fat, 2g protein & 5g carbs.

INGREDIENTS

- 1 can full-fat coconut milk
- 1 medium- or small-sized banana, ripe
- ½ tsp cinnamon
- 1 tsp vanilla extract
- ¼ cup chia seeds

INSTRUCTIONS

1. In a bowl, mash the banana until soft.
2. Add the remaining ingredients and mix until incorporated.
3. Cover and place in your refrigerator overnight.
4. Serve!

Strawberry Rhubarb Parfait

Prep + Cook Time: 1-2 days | Servings: 1

Amount per **one** serving: 449 cal., 45g fat, 6g protein & 6g carbs.

INGREDIENTS

- 1 package crème fraiche or plain full-fat yogurt (8.5 oz)
- 2 tbsp toasted almond flakes
- 2 tbsp toasted coconut flakes
- 6 tbsp homemade strawberry and rhubarb jam (4.25 oz)

INSTRUCTIONS

1. Add the jam into a dessert bowl (3 tbsp per serving).
2. Add the crème fraîche and garnish with the toasted almond and coconut flakes.
3. Serve!

Sausage Egg Muffins

Prep + Cook Time: 30 minutes | Servings: 4

Amount per **one** serving: 505 cal., 39g fat, 34g protein & 2g carbs.

INGREDIENTS

- 6 oz Italian sausage
- 6 eggs
- 1/8 cup heavy cream
- 3 oz cheese

INSTRUCTIONS

1. Preheat the oven to 350°F/175°C.
2. Grease a muffin pan.
3. Slice the sausage links and place them two to a tin.
4. Beat the eggs with the cream and season with salt and pepper.
5. Pour over the sausages in the tin.
6. Sprinkle with cheese and the remaining egg mixture.
7. Cook for 20 minutes or until the eggs are done and serve!

Salmon Omelet

Prep + Cook Time: 15 minutes | Servings: 2

Amount per **one** serving: 460 cal., 35g fat, 36g protein & 1.7g carbs.

INGREDIENTS

- 3 eggs
- 1 smoked salmon
- 3 links pork sausage
- ¼ cup onions
- ¼ cup provolone cheese

INSTRUCTIONS

1. Whisk the eggs and pour them into a skillet.
2. Follow the standard method for making an omelette.
3. Add the onions, salmon and cheese before turning the omelet over.
4. Sprinkle the omelet with cheese and serve with the sausages on the side.
5. Serve!

Egg Parmesan Breakfast Casserole

Prep + Cook Time: 40 minutes | Servings: 4

Amount per **one** serving: 475 cal., 45g fat, 38g protein & 2.5g carbs.

INGREDIENTS

- 5 eggs
- 3 tbsp chunky tomato sauce
- 2 tbsp heavy cream
- 2 tbsp grated parmesan cheese

INSTRUCTIONS

1. Preheat your oven to 350°F/175°C.
2. Combine the eggs and cream in a bowl.
3. Mix in the tomato sauce and add the cheese.
4. Spread into a glass baking dish and bake for 25-35 minutes.
5. Top with extra cheese.
6. Enjoy!

Hash Browns

Prep + Cook Time: 30 minutes | Servings: 4

Amount per **one** serving: 120 cal., 9g fat, 9g protein & 3g carbs.

INGREDIENTS

- 12 oz grated fresh cauliflower (about ½ a medium-sized head)
- 4 slices bacon, chopped
- 3 oz onion, chopped
- 1 tbsp butter, softened

INSTRUCTIONS

1. In a skillet, sauté the bacon and onion until brown.
2. Add in the cauliflower and stir until tender and browned.
3. Add the butter steadily as it cooks.
4. Season to taste with salt and pepper.
5. Enjoy!

Bacon Cups

Prep + Cook Time: 30 minutes | Servings: 2

Amount per **one** serving: 205 cal., 15g fat, 14g protein & 1g carbs.

INGREDIENTS

- 2 eggs
- 1 slice tomato
- 3 slices bacon
- 2 slices ham
- 2 tsp grated parmesan cheese

INSTRUCTIONS

1. Preheat your oven to 375°F/190°C.
2. Cook the bacon for half of the directed time.
3. Slice the bacon strips in half and line 2 greased muffin tins with 3 half-strips of bacon
4. Put one slice of ham and half slice of tomato in each muffin tin on top of the bacon
5. Crack one egg on top of the tomato in each muffin tin and sprinkle each with half a teaspoon of grated parmesan cheese.
6. Bake for 20 minutes.
7. Remove and let cool.
8. Serve!

Spinach Eggs & Cheese

Prep + Cook Time: 40 minutes | Servings: 3

Amount per **one** serving: 200 cal., 25g fat, 16g protein & 2g carbs.

INGREDIENTS

- 3 whole eggs
- 3 oz cottage cheese
- 3-4 oz chopped spinach
- ¼ cup parmesan cheese
- ¼ cup of milk

INSTRUCTIONS

1. Preheat your oven to 375°F/190°C.
2. In a large bowl, whisk the eggs, cottage cheese, the parmesan and the milk.
3. Mix in the spinach.
4. Transfer to a small, greased, oven dish.
5. Sprinkle the cheese on top.
6. Bake for 25-30 minutes.
7. Let cool for 5 minutes and serve.
8. Serve!

Fried Eggs

Prep + Cook Time: 8 minutes | Servings: 1

Amount per **one** serving: 220 cal., 21g fat, 12g protein & 1g carbs.

INGREDIENTS

- 2 eggs
- 3 slices bacon

INSTRUCTIONS

1. Heat some oil in a deep fryer at 375°F/190°C.
2. Fry the bacon.
3. In a small bowl, add the 2 eggs.
4. Quickly add the eggs into the center of the fryer.
5. Using two spatulas, form the egg into a ball while frying.
6. Fry for 2-3 minutes, until it stops bubbling.
7. Place on a paper towel and allow to drain.
8. Enjoy!

Scotch Eggs

Prep + Cook Time: 35 minutes | Servings: 2

Amount per **one** serving: 345 cal., 28g fat, 18g protein & 2g carbs.

INGREDIENTS

- 4 large eggs
- 1 package Jimmy Dean's Pork Sausage (12 oz)
- 8 slices thick-cut bacon
- 4 toothpicks

INSTRUCTIONS

1. Hard-boil the eggs, peel the shells and let them cool.
2. Slice the sausage into four parts and place each part into a large circle.
3. Put an egg into each circle and wrap it in the sausage.
4. Place inside your refrigerator for 1 hour.
5. Make a cross with two pieces of thick-cut bacon.
6. Place a wrapped egg in the center, fold the bacon over top of the egg and secure with a toothpick.
7. Cook inside your oven at 450°F/230°C for 25 minutes.
8. Enjoy!

Breakfast Cheesy Sausage

Serves: 2 | Prep Time: 20 mins

INGREDIENTS

- Pork sausage links, cut open and casing discarded
- Sea salt & Black pepper
- ½ teaspoon thyme
- ½ teaspoon sage
- 1 cup shredded mozzarella cheese

INSTRUCTIONS

1 Add the sea salt, sausage meat, thyme, black pepper, mozzarella cheese and sage into a bowl and mix well.

2 Form 2 equal patties out of the mixture and cook on a hot pan for 5 minutes each side.

3 Serve!

Nutrition Amount per serving

Calories 244, Total Fat 19.5g 25%, Saturated Fat 7g 35%, Cholesterol 59mg 19%, Sodium 651mg 28%, Total Carbs 0.75g 0%, Dietary Fiber 0.1g 1%, Protein 15.5g

Cauliflower Toast & Avocado

Serves: 2 | Prep Time: 20 mins

INGREDIENTS

- 1 large egg
- 1 grated cauliflower head
- 1 chopped avocado
- ¾ cup shredded mozzarella cheese
- Salt & Black pepper

INSTRUCTIONS

1 Set the oven to preheat at 4200 F then line the baking tray with a parchment paper

2 Cook the cauliflower in the microwave on high for 7 minutes

3 Allow the cauliflower to cool then drain on paper towel.

4 Remove the excess moisture by pressing with a clean kitchen towel then put them in a bowl.

5 Add the egg and mozzarella then stir

6 Add the seasonings and mix evenly then shape the mixture into medium squares

7 Arrange the squares on the prepared baking tray.

8 Allow to bake until browned evenly, for about 20 minutes

9 In the meantime, puree the avocado with black pepper and salt.

10 Top with the pureed avocado.

11 Serve!

Nutrition Amount per serving

Calories 126, Total Fat 6.5g 9%, Saturated Fat 2.3g 12%, Cholesterol 98mg 33%, Sodium 138mg 6%, Total Carbs 9.2g 3%, Dietary Fiber 4.7g 17%, Protein 9.2g

Millennials' Keto Avocado Toast

Serves: 2 | Prep Time: 20 mins

INGREDIENTS

- tablespoons sunflower oil
- ½ cup shredded parmesan cheese
- 1 sliced avocado
- Sea salt
- 4 slices cauliflower bread

INSTRUCTIONS

1 Pour the oil in a pan to heat then fry the cauliflower bread slices for 2 minutes each side.

2 Sprinkle the seasonings on the avocado and place on the cauliflower bread topped with the cheese.

3 Cook in the microwave for 2 minutes.

4 Serve!

Nutrition Amount per serving

Calories 140, Total Fat 11g13%, Saturated, Fat 4.5g 23%, Cholesterol 21mg 7%, Sodium 386mg 17%, Total Carbs 4.6g 2%, Dietary Fiber 2.3g 9%, Total Sugars 0.75g, Protein 10.6g

Chocolate Chip Waffles

Serves: 2 | Prep Time: 30 mins

INGREDIENTS

- scoops vanilla protein powder
- 1 teaspoon sea salt
- 50 grams sugar-free chocolate chips
- 2 large eggs
- 2 tablespoons melted butter

INSTRUCTIONS

1 Put the butter, vanilla protein powder and egg yolks in a bowl and mix well.

2 In another bowl, whisk the egg whites thoroughly then add to the vanilla mixture.

3 Gently fold in the chocolate chips and salt.

4 Cook the mixture on the waffle maker in relation to manufacturer's guidelines.

5 Serve!

Nutrition Amount per serving

Calories 300, Total Fat 18.7g 24%, Saturated Fat 9.6g 49%, Cholesterol 228mg 76%, Sodium 241mg 11%, Total Carbs 6.8g 3%, Dietary Fiber 1.2g 4%, Total Sugars 1.3g, Protein 29.8g

Egg Crepes with Avocados

Serves: 2 | Prep Time: 15 mins

INGREDIENTS

- 4 eggs
- ¾ sliced avocado
- 2 teaspoons olive oil
- ½ cup alfalfa sprouts
- 4 slices shredded turkey breast

INSTRUCTIONS

1 Pour the olive oil in a pan and heat over medium heat

2 Crush the eggs and cook for 3 minutes each side on the pan as you spread to cook evenly.

3 Remove the eggs from heat, then top with avocado, turkey breast, sprouts and alfalfa then roll up well.

4 Serve!

Nutrition Amount per serving

Calories 371, Total Fat 25.8g 33%, Saturated Fat 6g 30%, Cholesterol 363mg 121%, Sodium 1001mg 43%, Total Carbs 9.4g 3%, Dietary Fiber 4.5g 16%, Total Sugars 4g , Protein 27.1g

Ham and Cheese Pockets

Serves: 2 | Prep Time: 30 mins

INGREDIENTS

- 1 oz. cream cheese
- ¾ cup shredded mozzarella cheese
- 4 tablespoons flax meal
- 3 oz. provolone cheese slices
- 3 oz. ham

INSTRUCTIONS

1 Set the oven to preheat at 4000F then line a baking sheet with parchment paper.

2 Put the mozzarella cheese and cream cheese in a microwave to melt for 1 minute.

3 Add the flax meal to the melted mozzarella and mix well to form a dough.

4 Spread the dough and roll evenly

5 Top the provolone cheese slices and ham on the rolled dough

6 Shape the dough into an envelope-like shape.

7 Close the edges and make some holes in it.

8 Arrange them well on the baking tray and put in the oven.

9 Allow baking for 20 minutes then remove from the oven to cool.

10 Slice halt way.

11 Serve!

Nutrition Amount per serving

Calories 360, Total Fat 27.5g 35%, Saturated Fat 13.2g 65%, Cholesterol 81mg 28%, Sodium 834mg 36%, Total Carbs 7.8g 3%, Dietary Fiber 45g 16%, Total Sugars 0g , Protein 24.3g

Clementine and Pistachio Ricotta

Serves: 2 | Prep Time: 10 mins

INGREDIENTS

- teaspoons chopped pistachios
- ¾ cup ricotta
- 4 strawberries
- 1 tablespoon melted butter
- 2 segmented clementine

INSTRUCTIONS

1 Have 2 serving bowls then put equal amounts of ricotta in each bowl.

2 Add the strawberries, butter, pistachios and clementine segments to serve.

3 Serve!

Nutrition Amount per serving

Calories 311, Total Fat 25.1g 32%, Saturated Fat 15.1g 76%, Cholesterol 71mg 24%, Sodium 243mg 11%, Total Carbs 12.7g 5%, Dietary Fiber 1.2g 4%, Total Sugars 7.1g, Protein 10.7g

SNACKS

"I don't go long without eating. I never starve myself: I grab a healthy snack."

Chipotle Jicama Hash

Prep + Cook Time: 15 minutes | Servings: 2

Amount per **one** serving: 265 cal., 23g fat, 19g protein & 11g carbs.

INGREDIENTS

- 4 slices bacon, chopped
- 12 oz jicama, peeled and diced
- 4 oz purple onion, chopped
- 1 oz green bell pepper (or poblano), seeded and chopped
- 4 tbsp Chipotle mayonnaise

INSTRUCTIONS

1. Using a skillet, brown the bacon on a high heat.
2. Remove and place on a towel to drain the grease.
3. Use the remaining grease to fry the onions and jicama until brown.
4. When ready, add the bell pepper and cook the hash until tender.
5. Transfer the hash onto two plates and serve each plate with 4 tablespoons of Chipotle mayonnaise.

Fried Queso Blanco

Prep + Cook Time: 170 minutes | Servings: 4

Amount per **one** serving: 307 cal., 24g fat, 17g protein & 3g carbs.

INGREDIENTS

- 5 oz queso blanco
- 1 ½ tbsp olive oil
- 3 oz cheese
- 2 oz olives
- 1 pinch red pepper flakes

INSTRUCTIONS

1. Cube some cheese and freeze it for 1-2 hours.
2. Pour the oil in a skillet and heat to boil over a medium temperature.
3. Add the cheese cubes and heat till brown.
4. Combine the cheese together using a spatula and flatten.
5. Cook the cheese on both sides, flipping regularly.
6. While flipping, fold the cheese into itself to form crispy layers.
7. Use a spatula to roll it into a block.
8. Remove it from the pan, allow it to cool, cut it into small cubes, and serve.

Spinach with Bacon & Shallots

Prep + Cook Time: 30 minutes | Servings: 4

Amount per **one** serving: 150 cal., 13g fat, 4g protein & 5g carbs.

INGREDIENTS

- 16 oz raw spinach
- ½ cup chopped white onion
- ½ cup chopped shallot
- ½ pound raw bacon slices
- 2 tbsp butter

INSTRUCTIONS

1. Slice the bacon strips into small narrow pieces.
2. In a skillet, heat the butter and add the chopped onion, shallots and bacon.
3. Sauté for 15-20 minutes or until the onions start to caramelize and the bacon is cooked.
4. Add the spinach and sauté on a medium heat. Stir frequently to ensure the leaves touch the skillet while cooking.
5. Cover and steam for around 5 minutes, stir and continue until wilted.
6. Serve!

Bacon-Wrapped Sausage Skewers

Prep + Cook Time: 8 minutes | Servings: 2

Amount per **one** serving: 290 cal., 22g fat, 8g protein & 1g carbs.

INGREDIENTS
- 5 Italian chicken sausages
- 10 slices bacon

INSTRUCTIONS
1. Preheat your deep fryer to 370°F/190°C.
2. Cut the sausage into four pieces.
3. Slice the bacon in half.
4. Wrap the bacon over the sausage.
5. Skewer the sausage.
6. Fry for 4-5 minutes until browned.

Roasted Brussels Sprouts & Bacon

Prep + Cook Time: 45 minutes | Servings: 2

Amount per **one** serving: 130 cal., 9g fat, 7g protein & 5g carbs.

INGREDIENTS
- 24 oz brussels sprouts
- ¼ cup fish sauce
- ¼ cup bacon grease
- 6 strips bacon
- Pepper to taste

INSTRUCTIONS
1. De-stem and quarter the brussels sprouts.
2. Mix them with the bacon grease and fish sauce.
3. Slice the bacon into small strips and cook.
4. Add the bacon and pepper to the sprouts.
5. Spread onto a greased pan and cook at 450°F/230°C for 35 minutes.
6. Stir every 5 minute or so.
7. Broil for a few more minutes and serve.

Ham & Cheese Rolls

Prep + Cook Time: 5 minutes | Servings: 4

Amount per **one** serving: 200 cal., 12g fat, 16g protein & 3g carbs.

INGREDIENTS

- 16 slices ham
- 1 package chive and onion cream cheese (8 oz)
- 16 slices thin Swiss cheese

INSTRUCTIONS

1. Place the ham on a chopping board.
2. Dry the slices with a paper towel.
3. Thinly spread 2 teaspoons of Swiss cheese over each slice of ham.
4. On the clean section of ham, add a half inch slice of cheese.
5. On the cheese side, fold the ham over the cheese and roll it up.
6. Leave it as is, or slice into smaller rolls.

Hillbilly Cheese Surprise

Prep + Cook Time: 40 minutes | Servings: 6

Amount per **one** serving: 436 cal., 38g fat, 12g protein & 4g carbs.

INGREDIENTS

- 4 cups broccoli florets
- ¼ cup ranch dressing
- ½ cup sharp cheddar cheese, shredded
- ¼ cup heavy whipping cream
- Kosher salt and pepper to taste

INSTRUCTIONS

1. Preheat your oven to 375°F/190°C.
2. In a bowl, combine all of the ingredients until the broccoli is well-covered.
3. In a casserole dish, spread out the broccoli mixture.
4. Bake for 30 minutes.
5. Take out of your oven and mix.
6. If the florets are not tender, bake for another 5 minutes until tender.
7. Serve!

Parmesan & Garlic Cauliflower

Prep + Cook Time: 40 minutes | Servings: 4

Amount per **one** serving: 180 cal., 18g fat, 7g protein & 6g carbs.

INGREDIENTS

- 3/4 cup cauliflower florets
- 2 tbsp butter
- 1 clove garlic, sliced thinly
- 2 tbsp shredded parmesan
- 1 pinch of salt

INSTRUCTIONS

1. Preheat your oven to 350°F/175°C.
2. On a low heat, melt the butter with the garlic for 5-10 minutes.
3. Strain the garlic in a sieve.
4. Add the cauliflower, parmesan and salt.
5. Bake for 20 minutes or until golden.

Jalapeño Guacamole

Prep + Cook Time: 30 minutes | Servings: 4

Amount per **one** serving: 130 cal., 10g fat, 3g protein & 9g carbs.

INGREDIENTS

- 2 Hass avocados, ripe
- ¼ red onion
- 1 jalapeño
- 1 tbsp fresh lime juice
- Sea salt

INSTRUCTIONS

1. Spoon the avocado innings into a bowl.
2. Dice the jalapeño and onion.
3. Mash the avocado to the desired consistency.
4. Add in the onion, jalapeño and lime juice.
5. Sprinkle with salt.

Green Beans & Almonds

Prep + Cook Time: 15 minutes | Servings: 4

Amount per **one** serving: 178 cal., 16g fat, 4g protein & 4g carbs.

INGREDIENTS

- 1 lb fresh green beans, trimmed
- 2 tbsp butter
- ¼ cup sliced almonds
- 2 tsp lemon pepper

INSTRUCTIONS

1. Steam the green beans for 8 minutes, until tender, then drain.
2. On a medium heat, melt the butter in a skillet.
3. Sauté the almonds until browned.
4. Sprinkle with salt and pepper.
5. Mix in the green beans.

Sugar Snap Bacon

Prep + Cook Time: 10 minutes | Servings: 4

Amount per **one** serving: 80 cal., 4g fat, 3g protein & 1g carbs.

INGREDIENTS

- 3 cups sugar snap peas
- ½ tbsp lemon juice
- 2 tbsp bacon fat
- 2 tsp garlic
- ½ tsp red pepper flakes

INSTRUCTIONS

1. In a skillet, cook the bacon fat until it begins to smoke.
2. Add the garlic and cook for 2 minutes.
3. Add the sugar peas and lemon juice.
4. Cook for 2-3 minutes.
5. Remove and sprinkle with red pepper flakes and lemon zest.
6. Serve!

Flax Cheese Chips

Prep + Cook Time: 20 minutes | Servings: 2

Amount per **one** serving: 130 cal., 8g fat, 5g protein & 1g carbs.

INGREDIENTS

- 1 ½ cup cheddar cheese
- 4 tbsp ground flaxseed meal
- Seasonings of your choice

INSTRUCTIONS

1. Preheat your oven to 425°F/220°C.
2. Spoon 2 tablespoons of cheddar cheese into a mound, onto a non-stick pad.
3. Spread out a pinch of flax seed on each chip.
4. Season and bake for 10-15 minutes.

Country Style Chard

Prep + Cook Time: 5 minutes | Servings: 2

Amount per **one** serving: 190 cal., 4g fat, 5g protein & 10g carbs.

INGREDIENTS

- 4 slices bacon, chopped
- 2 tbsp butter
- 2 tbsp fresh lemon juice
- ½ tsp garlic paste
- 1 bunch Swiss chard, stems removed, leaves cut into 1-inch pieces

INSTRUCTIONS

1. On a medium heat, cook the bacon in a skillet until the fat begins to brown.
2. Melt the butter in the skillet and add the lemon juice and garlic paste.
3. Add the chard leaves and cook until they begin to wilt.
4. Cover and turn up the heat to high.
5. Cook for 3 minutes.
6. Mix well, sprinkle with salt and serve.

Kale Crisps

Prep + Cook Time: 15 minutes | Servings: 1

Amount per **one** serving: 60 cal., 3g fat, 2g protein & 2g carbs.

INGREDIENTS

- 1 large bunch kale
- 2 tbsp olive oil
- 1 tbsp seasoned salt

INSTRUCTIONS

1. Preheat your oven to 350°F/175°C.
2. De-stem, wash and dry the kale.
3. Put it inside a Ziploc bag and shake with oil.
4. Put the kale on a baking sheet.
5. Bake for 10 minutes.
6. Remove and serve hot!

Baked Tortillas

Prep + Cook Time: 30 minutes | Servings: 4

Amount per **one** serving: 89 cal., 6g fat, 3g protein & 4g carbs.

INGREDIENTS

- 1 large head of cauliflower, divided into florets.
- 4 large eggs
- 2 garlic cloves (minced)
- 1 ½ tsp herbs (whatever your favorite is - basil, oregano, thyme)
- ½ tsp salt

INSTRUCTIONS

1. Preheat your oven to 375°F/190°C.
2. Put parchment paper on two baking sheets.
3. In a food processor, break down the cauliflower into rice.
4. Add ¼ cup water and the riced cauliflower to a saucepan.
5. Cook on a medium high heat until tender for 10 minutes. Drain.
6. Dry with a clean kitchen towel.
7. Mix the cauliflower, eggs, garlic, herbs and salt.
8. Make 4 thin circles on the parchment paper.
9. Bake for 20 minutes, until dry.

Homemade Mayonnaise

Prep + Cook Time: 30 minutes | Servings: 4

Amount per **one** serving: 95 cal., 9g fat, 9g protein & 1g carbs.

INGREDIENTS

- 1 large egg
- Juice from 1 lemon.
- 1 tsp dry mustard
- ½ tsp black pepper
- 1 cup avocado oil

INSTRUCTIONS

1. Combine the egg and lemon juice in a container and let sit for 20 minutes.
2. Add the dry mustard, pepper, and avocado oil.
3. Insert an electric whisk into the container.
4. Blend for 30 seconds.
5. Transfer to a sealed container and store in your refrigerator.

Hollandaise Sauce

Prep + Cook Time: 2 minutes | Servings: 8

Amount per **one** serving: 95 cal., 50g fat, 3g protein & 1g carbs.

INGREDIENTS

- 8 large emulsified egg yolks
- ½ tsp salt
- 2 tbsp fresh lemon juice
- 1 cup unsalted butter

INSTRUCTIONS

1. Combine the egg yolks, salt, and lemon juice in a blender until smooth.
2. Put the butter in your microwave for around 60 seconds, until melted and hot.
3. Turn the blender on a low speed and slowly pour in the butter until the sauce begins to thicken.
4. Serve!

Garlicky Green Beans

Prep + Cook Time: 10 minutes | Servings: 4

Amount per **one** serving: 215 cal., 9g fat, 4g protein & 7g carbs.

INGREDIENTS

- 1 lb green beans, trimmed
- 1 cup butter
- 2 cloves garlic, minced
- 1 cup toasted pine nuts

INSTRUCTIONS

1. Boil a pot of water.
2. Add the green beans and cook until tender for 5 minutes.
3. Heat the butter in a large skillet over a high heat. Add the garlic and pine nuts and sauté for 2 minutes or until the pine nuts are lightly browned.
4. Transfer the green beans to the skillet and turn until coated.
5. Serve!

MEALS

"I love spending time with my friends and family. The simplest things in life give me the most pleasure: cooking a good meal, enjoying my friends."

Monkey Salad

Prep + Cook Time: 10 minutes | Servings: 12

Amount per **one** serving: 240 cal., 22g fat, 4g protein & 4g carbs.

INGREDIENTS

- 2 tbsp butter
- 1 cup unsweetened coconut flakes
- 1 cup raw, unsalted cashews
- 1 cup raw, unsalted almonds
- 1 cup 90% dark chocolate shavings

INSTRUCTIONS

1.   In a skillet, melt the butter on a medium heat.
2.   Add the coconut flakes and sauté until lightly browned for 4 minutes.
3.   Add the cashews and almonds and sauté for 3 minutes. Remove from the heat and sprinkle with dark chocolate shavings.
4.   Serve!

Jarlsberg Lunch Omelet

Prep + Cook Time: 10 minutes | Servings: 2

Amount per **one** serving: 525 cal., 37g fat, 40g protein & 2g carbs.

INGREDIENTS

- 4 medium mushrooms, sliced, 2 oz
- 1 green onion, sliced
- 2 eggs, beaten
- 1 oz Jarlsberg or Swiss cheese, shredded
- 1 oz ham, diced

INSTRUCTIONS

1. In a skillet, cook the mushrooms and green onion until tender.
2. Add the eggs and mix well.
3. Sprinkle with salt and top with the mushroom mixture, cheese and the ham.
4. When the egg is set, fold the plain side of the omelet on the filled side.
5. Turn off the heat and let it stand until the cheese has melted.
6. Serve!

Mu Shu Lunch Pork

Prep + Cook Time: 10 minutes | Servings: 4

Amount per **one** serving: 260 cal., 10g fat, 30g protein & 10g carbs.

INGREDIENTS

- 4 cups coleslaw mix, with carrots
- 1 small onion, sliced thin
- 1 lb cooked roast pork, cut into ½" cubes
- 2 tbsp hoisin sauce
- 2 tbsp soy sauce

INSTRUCTIONS

1. In a large skillet, heat the oil on a high heat.
2. Stir-fry the cabbage and onion for 4 minutes until tender.
3. Add the pork, hoisin and soy sauce.
4. Cook until browned.
5. Enjoy!

Fiery Jalapeno Poppers

Prep + Cook Time: 40 minutes | Servings: 4

Amount per **one** serving: 550 cal., 12g fat, 25g protein & 5g carbs.

INGREDIENTS

- 5 oz cream cheese
- ¼ cup mozzarella cheese
- 8 medium jalapeno peppers
- ½ tsp Mrs. Dash Table Blend
- 8 slices bacon

INSTRUCTIONS

1. Preheat your oven to 400°F/200°C.
2. Cut the jalapenos in half.
3. Use a spoon to scrape out the insides of the peppers.
4. In a bowl, add together the cream cheese, mozzarella cheese and spices of your choice.
5. Pack the cream cheese mixture into the jalapenos and place the peppers on top.
6. Wrap each pepper in 1 slice of bacon, starting from the bottom and working up.
7. Bake for 30 minutes. Broil for an additional 3 minutes.
8. Serve!

Bacon & Chicken Patties

Prep + Cook Time: 15 minutes | Servings: 2

Amount per **one** serving: 420 cal., 22g fat, 37g protein & 4g carbs.

INGREDIENTS

- 1 ½ oz can chicken breast
- 4 slices bacon
- ¼ cup parmesan cheese
- 1 large egg
- 3 tbsp keto coconut flour

INSTRUCTIONS

1. Cook the bacon until crispy.
2. Chop the chicken and bacon together in a food processor until fine.
3. Add in the parmesan, egg, coconut flour and mix.
4. Make the patties by hand and fry on a medium heat in a pan with some oil.
5. Once browned, flip over, continue cooking, and lie them to drain.
6. Serve!

Cheddar Bacon Burst

Prep + Cook Time: 90 minutes | Servings: 8

Amount per **one** serving: 430 cal., 33g fat, 26g protein & 3g carbs.

INGREDIENTS

- 30 slices bacon
- 2 ½ cups cheddar cheese
- 4-5 cups raw spinach
- 1-2 tbsp Tones Southwest Chipotle Seasoning
- 2 tsp Mrs. Dash Table Seasoning

INSTRUCTIONS

1. Preheat your oven to 375°F/190°C.
2. Weave the bacon into 15 vertical pieces & 12 horizontal pieces. Cut the extra 3 in half to fill in the rest, horizontally.
3. Season the bacon.
4. Add the cheese to the bacon.
5. Add the spinach and press down to compress.
6. Tightly roll up the woven bacon.
7. Line a baking sheet with kitchen foil and add plenty of salt to it.
8. Put the bacon on top of a cooling rack and put that on top of your baking sheet.
9. Bake for 60-70 minutes.
10. Let cool for 10-15 minutes before
11. Slice and enjoy!

Grilled Ham & Cheese

Prep + Cook Time: 30 minutes | Servings: 3

Amount per **one** serving: 230 cal., 21g fat, 15g protein & 2g carbs.

INGREDIENTS

- 3 low-carb buns
- 4 slices medium-cut deli ham
- 1 tbsp salted butter
- 3 slices cheddar cheese
- ½ cup almond flour
- 1 tsp. baking powder
- 2 eggs. Scrambled
- ½ tablespoon coconut flour

INSTRUCTIONS

Bread:

1. Preheat your oven to 350°F/175°C.
2. Mix the almond flour, salt and baking powder in a bowl. Put to the side.
3. Add in the butter and coconut oil to a skillet.
4. Melt for 20 seconds and pour into another bowl.
5. In this bowl, mix in the dough.
6. Scramble two eggs. Add to the dough.
7. Add ½ tablespoon of coconut flour to thicken, and place evenly into a cupcake tray. Fill about ¾ inch.
8. Bake for 20 minutes until browned.
9. Allow to cool for 15 minutes and cut each in half for the buns.

Sandwich:

1. Fry the deli meat in a skillet on a high heat.
2. Put the ham and cheese between the buns.
3. Heat the butter on medium high.
4. When brown, turn to low and add the dough to pan.
5. Press down with a weight until you smell burning, then flip to crisp both sides.
6. Enjoy!

Prosciutto Spinach Salad

Prep + Cook Time: 5 minutes | Servings: 2

Amount per **one** serving: 199 cal., 18g fat, 6.5g protein & 2.5g carbs.

INGREDIENTS

● 2 cups baby spinach

● 1/3 lb prosciutto

● 1 cantaloupe

● 1 avocado

● ¼ cup diced red onion handful of raw, unsalted walnuts

INSTRUCTIONS

1.   Put a cup of spinach on each plate.

2.   Top with the diced prosciutto, cubes of balls of melon, slices of avocado, a handful of red onion and a few walnuts.

3.   Add some freshly ground pepper, if you like.

4.   Serve!

Riced Cauliflower & Curry Chicken

Prep + Cook Time: 30 minutes | Servings: 6

Amount per **one** serving: 950 cal., 45g fat, 31g protein & 8g carbs.

INGREDIENTS

- 2 lbs chicken (4 breasts)
- 1 packet curry paste
- 3 tbsp ghee (can substitute with butter)
- ½ cup heavy cream
- 1 head cauliflower (around 1 kg)

INSTRUCTIONS

1. In a large skillet, melt the ghee.
2. Add the curry paste and mix.
3. Once combined, add a cup of water and simmer for 5 minutes.
4. Add the chicken, cover the skillet and simmer for 18 minutes.
5. Cut a cauliflower head into florets and blend in a food processor to make the riced cauliflower.
6. When the chicken is cooked, uncover, add the cream and cook for an additional 7 minutes.
7. Serve!

Mashed Garlic Turnips

Prep + Cook Time: 10 minutes | Servings: 2

Amount per **one** serving: 150 cal., 14g fat, 3g protein & 4g carbs.

INGREDIENTS

- 3 cups diced turnip
- 2 cloves garlic, minced
- ¼ cup heavy cream
- 3 tbsp melted butter
- Salt and pepper to season

INSTRUCTIONS

1. Boil the turnips until tender.
2. Drain and mash the turnips.
3. Add the cream, butter, salt, pepper and garlic. Combine well.
4. Serve!

Lasagna-Style Spaghetti Squash

Prep + Cook Time: 90 minutes | Servings: 6

Amount per **one** serving: 420 cal., 31g fat, 25g protein & 5g carbs.

INGREDIENTS

- 25 slices mozzarella cheese
- 1 large jar (40 oz) Rao's Marinara sauce
- 30 oz whole-milk ricotta cheese
- 2 large spaghetti squash, cooked (44 oz)
- 4 lbs ground beef

INSTRUCTIONS

1.   Preheat your oven to 375°F/190°C.
2.   Slice the spaghetti squash and place it face down inside an oven proof dish. Fill with water until covered.
3.   Bake for 45 minutes until skin is soft.
4.   Sear the meat until browned.
5.   In a large skillet, heat the browned meat and marinara sauce. Set aside when warm.
6.   Scrape the flesh off the cooked squash to resemble strands of spaghetti.
7.   Layer the lasagna in a large greased pan in alternating layers of spaghetti squash, meat sauce, mozzarella, ricotta. Repeat until all increased have been used.
8.   Bake for an 30 minutes and serve!

Blue Cheese Chicken Wedges

Prep + Cook Time: 45 minutes | Servings: 4

Amount per **one** serving: 315 cal., 22g fat, 19g protein & 8g carbs.

INGREDIENTS

- Blue cheese dressing
- 2 tbsp crumbled blue cheese
- 4 strips of bacon
- 2 chicken breasts (boneless)
- 3/4 cup of your favorite buffalo sauce

INSTRUCTIONS

1. Boil a large pot of salted water.
2. Add in two chicken breasts to pot and cook for 28 minutes.
3. Turn off the heat and let the chicken rest for 10 minutes. Using a fork, pull the chicken apart into strips.
4. Cook and cool the bacon strips, and put to the side.
5. On a medium heat, combine the chicken and buffalo sauce. Stir until hot.
6. Add the blue cheese and buffalo pulled chicken. Top with the cooked bacon crumble.
7. Serve and enjoy.

'Oh, so good' Salad

Prep + Cook Time: 10 minutes | Servings: 2

Amount per **one** serving: 110 cal., 10g fat, 4g protein & 2g carbs.

INGREDIENTS

- 6 brussels sprouts
- ½ tsp apple cider vinegar
- 1 tsp olive/grapeseed oil
- 1 grind of salt
- 1 tbsp freshly grated parmesan

INSTRUCTIONS

1. Slice the clean brussels sprouts in half.
2. Cut thin slices in the opposite direction.
3. Once sliced, cut the roots off and discard.
4. Toss together with the apple cider, oil and salt.
5. Sprinkle with the parmesan cheese, combine and enjoy!

I Love Bacon

Prep + Cook Time: 90 minutes | Servings: 4

Amount per **one** serving: 388 cal., 38g fat, 29g protein & 3g carbs.

INGREDIENTS

- 30 slices thick-cut bacon
- 12 oz steak
- 10 oz pork sausage
- 4 oz cheddar cheese, shredded

INSTRUCTIONS

1. Lay out 5 x 6 slices of bacon in a woven pattern and bake at 400°F/200°C for 20 minutes until crisp.
2. Combine the steak, bacon and sausage to form a meaty mixture.
3. Lay out the meat in a rectangle of similar size to the bacon strips. Season with salt/peppe.
4. Place the bacon weave on top of the meat mixture.
5. Place the cheese in the center of the bacon.
6. Roll the meat into a tight roll and refrigerate.
7. Make a 7 x 7 bacon weave and roll the bacon weave over the meat, diagonally.
8. Bake at 400°F/200°C for 60 minutes or 165°F/75°C internally.
9. Let rest for 5 minutes before serving.

Lemon Dill Trout

Prep + Cook Time: 10 minutes | Servings: 1

Amount per **one** serving: 460 cal., 22g fat, 57g protein & 1g carbs.

INGREDIENTS

- 2 lb pan-dressed trout (or other small fish), fresh or frozen
- 1 ½ tsp salt
- ½ cup butter or margarine
- 2 tbsp dill weed
- 3 tbsp lemon juice

INSTRUCTIONS

1. Cut the fish lengthwise and season the with pepper.
2. Prepare a skillet by melting the butter and dill weed.
3. Fry the fish on a high heat, flesh side down, for 2-3 minutes per side.
4. Remove the fish. Add the lemon juice to the butter and dill to create a sauce.
5. Serve the fish with the sauce.

No Potato Shepherd's Pie

Prep + Cook Time: 70 minutes | Servings: 6

Amount per **one** serving: 480 cal., 28g fat, 12g protein & 10g carbs.

INGREDIENTS

- ●1 lb lean ground beef
- ●8 oz low-carb mushroom sauce mix
- ●¼ cup ketchup
- ●1 lb package frozen mixed vegetables
- ●1 lb Aitkin's low-carb bake mix or equivalent

INSTRUCTIONS

1.   Preheat your oven to 375°F/190°C.

2.   Prepare the bake mix according to package instructions. Layer into the skillet base.

3.   Brown the ground beef with the salt. Stir in the mushroom sauce, ketchup and mixed vegetables.

4.   Bring the mixture to the boil and reduce the heat to medium, cover and simmer until tender.

5.   Bake until piping hot and serve!

Easy Slider

Prep + Cook Time: 70 minutes | Servings: 6

Amount per **one** serving: 419 cal., 35g fat, 20g protein & 8g carbs.

INGREDIENTS

- ½ lb Ground Beef
- 5 Eggs
- Garlic/salt/pepper/onion powder to taste
- Several dashes of Worcestershire sauce
- 8 oz cheddar cheese (½ oz per patty)

INSTRUCTIONS

1. Mix the beef, eggs and spices together.
2. Divide the meat into 1.5 oz patties.
3. Add a half-ounce of cheese to each patty and combine two patties to make one burger, like a sandwich. Heat the oil on high and fry the burgers until cooked as desired. Serve.

Dijon Halibut Steak

Prep + Cook Time: 20 minutes | Servings: 1

Amount per **one** serving: 305 cal., 16g fat, 34g protein & 6g carbs.

INGREDIENTS

- 1 6-oz fresh or thawed halibut steak
- 1 tbsp butter
- 1 tbsp lemon juice
- ½ tbsp Dijon mustard
- 1 tsp fresh basil

INSTRUCTIONS

1. Heat the butter, basil, lemon juice and mustard in a small saucepan to make a glaze.
2. Brush both sides of the halibut steak with the mixture.
3. Grill the fish for 10 minutes over a medium heat until tender and flakey.

Cast-Iron Cheesy Chicken

Prep + Cook Time: 10 minutes | Servings: 4

Amount per **one** serving: 419 cal., 29g fat, 32g protein & 2g carbs.

INGREDIENTS

- 4 chicken breasts
- 4 bacon strips
- 4 oz ranch dressing
- 2 green onions
- 4 oz cheddar cheese

INSTRUCTIONS

1. Pour the oil into a skillet and heat on high. Add the chicken breasts and fry both sides until piping hot.
2. Fry the bacon and crumble it into bits.
3. Dice the green onions.
4. Put the chicken in a baking dish and top with soy sauce.
5. Toss in the ranch, bacon, green onions and top with cheese.
6. Cook until the cheese is browned, for around 4 minutes.
7. Serve.

Cauliflower Rice Chicken Curry

Prep + Cook Time: 40 minutes | Servings: 4

Amount per **one** serving: 249 cal., 18g fat, 15g protein & 6g carbs.

INGREDIENTS

- 2 lb chicken (4 breasts)
- 1 packet curry paste
- 3 tbsp ghee (can substitute with butter)
- ½ cup heavy cream
- 1 head cauliflower (around 1 kg/2.2 lb)

INSTRUCTIONS

1. Melt the ghee in a pot. Mix in the curry paste.
2. Add the water and simmer for 5 minutes.
3. Add the chicken, cover, and simmer on a medium heat for 20 minutes or until the chicken is cooked.
4. Shred the cauliflower florets in a food processor to resemble rice.
5. Once the chicken is cooked, uncover, and incorporate the cream.
6. Cook for 7 minutes and serve over the cauliflower.

Bacon Chops

Prep + Cook Time: 20 minutes | Servings: 2

Amount per **one** serving: 439 cal., 39g fat, 12g protein & 9g carbs.

INGREDIENTS

- 2 pork chops (I prefer bone-in, but boneless chops work great as well)
- 1 bag shredded brussels sprouts
- 4 slices of bacon
- Worcestershire sauce
- Lemon juice (optional)

INSTRUCTIONS

1.   Place the pork chops on a baking sheet with the Worcestershire sauce inside a preheated grill for 5 minutes.

2.   Turnover and cook for another 5 minutes. Put to the side when done.

3.   Cook the chopped bacon in a large pan until browned. Add the shredded brussels sprouts and cook together.

4.   Stir the brussels sprouts with the bacon and grease and cook for 5 minutes until the bacon is crisp.

Chicken in a Blanket

Prep + Cook Time: 60 minutes | Servings: 3

Amount per **one** serving: 380 cal., 29g fat, 11g protein & 3g carbs.

INGREDIENTS

- 3 boneless chicken breasts
- 1 package bacon
- 1 8-oz package cream cheese
- 3 jalapeno peppers
- Salt, pepper, garlic powder or other seasonings

INSTRUCTIONS

1. Cut the chicken breast in half lengthwise to create two pieces.
2. Cut the jalapenos in half lengthwise and remove the seeds.
3. Dress each breast with a half-inch slice of cream cheese and half a slice of jalapeno. Sprinkle with garlic powder, salt and pepper.
4. Roll the chicken and wrap 2 to 3 pieces of bacon around it—secure with toothpicks.
5. Bake in a preheated 375°F/190°C oven for 50 minutes.
6. Serve!

Stuffed Chicken Rolls

Prep + Cook Time: 45 minutes | Servings: 4

Amount per **one** serving: 270 cal., 11g fat, 38g protein & 1g carbs.

INGREDIENTS

- 4 boneless, skinless chicken breasts
- 7 oz cream cheese
- ¼ cup green onions, chopped
- 4 slices bacon, partially cooked

INSTRUCTIONS

1. Partially cook your strips of bacon, about 5 minutes for each side and set aside.
2. Pound the chicken breasts to a quarter-inch thick.
3. Mix the cream cheese and green onions together. Spread 2 tablespoons of the mixture onto each breast. Roll and wrap them with the strip of bacon, then secure with a toothpick.
4. Place the chicken on a baking sheet and bake in a preheated oven at 375°F/190°C for 30 minutes.
5. Broil for 5 minutes to crisp the bacon.
6. Serve.

Duck Fat Ribeye

Prep + Cook Time: 20 minutes | Servings: 1

Amount per **one** serving: 740 cal., 65g fat, 37g protein & 1g carbs

INGREDIENTS

- One 16-oz ribeye steak (1 - 1 ¼ inch thick)
- 1 tbsp duck fat (or other high smoke point oil like peanut oil)
- ½ tbsp butter
- ½ tsp thyme, chopped
- Salt and pepper to taste

INSTRUCTIONS

1.   Preheat a skillet in your oven at 400°F/200°C.
2.   Season the steaks with the oil, salt and pepper. Remove the skillet from the oven once pre-heated.
3.   Put the skillet on your stove top burner on a medium heat and drizzle in the oil.
4.   Sear the steak for 1-4 minutes, depending on if you like it rare, medium or well done.
5.   Turn over the steak and place in your oven for 6 minutes.
6.   Take out the steak from your oven and place it back on the stove top on low heat.
7.   Toss in the butter and thyme and cook for 3 minutes, basting as you go along.
8.   Rest for 5 minutes and serve.

Easy Zoodles & Turkey Balls

Prep + Cook Time: 35 minutes | Servings: 2

Amount per **one** serving: 287 cal., 14g fat, 24g protein & 10g carbs

INGREDIENTS

- 1 zucchini, cut into spirals
- 1 can vodka pasta sauce
- 1 package frozen Armour Turkey meatballs

INSTRUCTIONS

1. Cook the meatballs and sauce on a high heat for 25 minutes, stirring occasionally.
2. Wash the zucchini and put through a vegetable spiral maker.
3. Boil the water and blanch the raw zoodles for 60 seconds. Remove and drain.
4. Combine the zoodles and prepared saucy meatballs.
5. Serve!

Sausage Balls

Prep + Cook Time: 25 minutes | Servings: 6

Amount per **one** serving: 365 cal., 30g fat, 21g protein & 5g carbs

INGREDIENTS

- 12 oz Jimmy Dean's Sausage
- 6 oz. shredded cheddar cheese
- 10 cubes cheddar (optional)

INSTRUCTIONS

1. Mix the shredded cheese and sausage.
2. Divide the mixture into 12 equal parts to be stuffed.
3. Add a cube of cheese to the center of the sausage and roll into balls.
4. Fry at 375°F/190°C until crisp.
5. Serve!

Bacon Scallops Packages

Prep + Cook Time: 10 minutes | Servings: 6

Amount per **one** serving: 280 cal., 18g fat, 28g protein & 3g carbs

INGREDIENTS

● 12 scallops
● 12 thin bacon slices
● 12 toothpicks
● Salt and pepper to taste
● ½ tbsp oil

INSTRUCTIONS

1. Heat a skillet on a high heat while drizzling in the oil.
2. Wrap each scallop with a piece of thinly cut bacon—secure with a toothpick.
3. Season to taste.
4. Cook for 3 minutes per side.
5. Serve!

Gluten Free Gratin

Prep + Cook Time: 30 minutes | Servings: 2

Amount per **one** serving: 175 cal., 15g fat, 5g protein & 2g carbs

INGREDIENTS

- 4 cups raw cauliflower florets
- 4 tbsp butter
- 1/3 cup heavy whipping cream
- Salt and pepper to taste
- 5 deli slices pepper jack cheese

INSTRUCTIONS

1.   Combine the cauliflower, butter, cream, salt and pepper and microwave on medium for 20 minutes, or until tender.

2.   Mash with a fork. Season to your liking.

3.   Lay the slices of cheese across the top of the cauliflower.

4.   Cook inside your microwave for an additional 3 minutes, depending on the power of your microwave.

5.   Serve!

Buffalo Chicken Salad

Prep + Cook Time: 40 minutes | Servings: 1

Amount per **one** serving: 410 cal., 9g fat, 15g protein & 10g carbs

INGREDIENTS

- 3 cups salad of your choice
- 1 chicken breast
- 1/2 cup shredded cheese of your choice
- Buffalo wing sauce of your choice
- Ranch or blue cheese dressing

INSTRUCTIONS

1. Preheat your oven to 400°F/200°C.
2. Douse the chicken breast in the buffalo wing sauce and bake for 25 minutes. In the last 5 minutes, throw the cheese on the wings until it melts.
3. When cooked, remove from the oven and slice into pieces.
4. Place on a bed of lettuce.
5. Pour the salad dressing of your choice on top.
6. Serve!

Meatballs

Prep + Cook Time: 30 minutes | Servings: 6

Amount per **one** serving: 380 cal., 22g fat, 18g protein & 1g carbs

INGREDIENTS

- 1 lb ground beef (or ½ lb beef, ½ lb pork)
- ½ cup grated parmesan cheese
- 1 tbsp minced garlic (or paste)
- ½ cup mozzarella cheese
- 1 tsp freshly ground pepper

INSTRUCTIONS

1. Preheat your oven to 400°F/200°C.
2. In a bowl, mix all the ingredients together.
3. Roll the meat mixture into 6 generous meatballs.
4. Bake inside your oven at 170°F/80°C for about 18 minutes.
5. Serve with sauce!

Chicken Tenders

Prep + Cook Time: 40 minutes | Servings: 3

Amount per **one** serving: 340 cal., 25g fat, 20g protein & 2g carbs

INGREDIENTS

- 3 boneless, skinless chicken breasts (thawed)
- 1 4-oz bag spicy pork rinds/chicharrones
- 2 eggs

INSTRUCTIONS

1. Preheat your oven to 400°F/200°C.
2. Blend the pork rinds into small pieces and place onto a plate.
3. In a bowl, crack the eggs and whisk until mixed.
4. Slice the chicken breasts into 1x2 inch pieces.
5. One at a time, dip the pieces into the egg mixture and place on top of the crushed pork rinds.
6. Roll the pieces around until covered in the rind coating.
7. Put the chicken strips into an oven proof dish and bake for 28 minutes.
8. Serve!

Fat Bombs

Prep + Cook Time: 100 minutes | Servings: 2

Amount per **one** serving: 205 cal., 30g fat, 18g protein & 1g carbs

INGREDIENTS

- 1 cup coconut butter
- 1 cup coconut milk (full fat, canned)
- 1 tsp vanilla extract (gluten free)
- ½ tsp nutmeg
- ½ cup coconut shreds

INSTRUCTIONS

1. Pour some water into pot and put a glass bowl on top.
2. Add all the ingredients except the shredded coconut into the glass bowl and cook on a medium heat.
3. Stir and melt until they start melting.
4. Then, take them off of the heat.
5. Put the glass bowl into your refrigerator until the mix can be rolled into doughy balls. Usually this happens after around 30 minutes.
6. Roll the dough into 1-inch balls through the coconut shreds.
7. Place the balls on a plate and refrigerate for one hour.
8. Serve!

Beef Casserole

Prep + Cook Time: 40 minutes | Servings: 2

Amount per **one** serving: 275 cal., 19g fat, 19g protein & 6g carbs

INGREDIENTS

- ½ lb ground beef
- ½ cup chopped onion
- ½ bag coleslaw mix
- 1-1/2 cups tomato sauce
- 1 tbsp lemon juice

INSTRUCTIONS

1. In a skillet, cook the ground beef until browned and to the side.
2. Mix in the onion and cabbage to the skillet and sauté until soft.
3. Add the ground beef back in along with the tomato sauce and lemon juice.
4. Bring the mixture to a boil, then cover and simmer for 30 minutes.
5. Enjoy!

Roast Beef Lettuce Wraps

Prep + Cook Time: 10 minutes | Servings: 4

Amount per **one** serving: 460 cal., 29g fat, 32g protein & 10g carbs

INGREDIENTS

- 8 large iceberg lettuce leaves
- 8 oz (8 slices) rare roast beef
- ½ cup homemade mayonnaise
- 8 slices provolone cheese
- 1 cup baby spinach

INSTRUCTIONS

1. Wash the lettuce leaves and sake them dry. Try not to rip them.
2. Place 1 slice of roast beef inside each wrap.
3. Smother 1 tablespoon of mayonnaise on top of each piece of roast beef.
4. Top the mayonnaise with 1 slice of provolone cheese and 1 cup of baby spinach.
5. Roll the lettuce up around the toppings.
6. Serve & enjoy!

Turkey Avocado Rolls

Prep + Cook Time: 10 minutes | Servings: 6

Amount per **one** serving: 150 cal., 9g fat, 15g protein & 5g carbs

INGREDIENTS

- 12 slices (12 oz) turkey breast
- 12 slices Swiss cheese
- 2 cups baby spinach
- 1 large avocado, cut into 12 slices
- 1 cup homemade mayonnaise

INSTRUCTIONS

1. Lay out the slices of turkey breast flat and place a slice of Swiss cheese on top of each one.
2. Top each slice with 1 cup baby spinach and 3 slices of avocado.
3. Drizzle the mayonnaise on top.
4. Sprinkle each "sandwich" with lemon pepper.
5. Roll up the sandwiches and secure with toothpicks.
6. Serve immediately or refrigerate until ready to serve.

'Nearly' Pizza

Prep + Cook Time: 30 minutes | Servings: 4

Amount per **one** serving: 420 cal., 34g fat, 26g protein & 10g carbs

INGREDIENTS

- 4 large portobello mushrooms
- 4 tsp olive oil
- 1 cup marinara sauce
- 1 cup shredded mozzarella cheese
- 10 slices sugar-free pepperoni

INSTRUCTIONS

1. Preheat your oven to 375°F/190°C.
2. De-steam the 4 mushrooms and brush each cap with the olive oil, one spoon for each cap.
3. Place on a baking sheet and bake stem side down for 8 minutes.
4. Take out of the oven and fill each cap with 1 cup marinara sauce, 1 cup mozzarella cheese and 3 slices of pepperoni.
5. Cook for another 10 minutes until browned.
6. Serve hot.

Cheesy Bacon Butternut Squash

Serves: 2 | Prep Time: 40 mins

INGREDIENTS

- 1 tablespoon olive oil
- ½ pound sliced butternut squash
- Kosher salt & Black pepper
- ½ cup grated Parmesan cheese
- 2 oz. chopped bacon

INSTRUCTIONS

1 Set the oven to 4250F to preheat then grease the baking tray

2 Add the olive oil in a medium skillet to heat to sauté the bacon, butternut squash, and the seasonings for 2 minutes.

3 After 2 minutes, pour everything on the baking tray to bake for 25 minutes

4 Remove from the oven, sprinkle the parmesan cheese on top the bake for 10 more minutes

5 Serve the meal while still warm.

Nutrition Amount per serving

Calories 335, Total Fat 23.7g 30%, Saturated Fat 7.2g 37%, Cholesterol 46mg 16%, Sodium 907mg 40%, Total Carbs 12g 5%, Dietary Fiber 2.1g 8%, Total Sugars 2.4g, Protein 19.3g

Jalapeño Popper Stuffed Zucchini

Serves: 2 | Prep Time: 30 mins

INGREDIENTS

- ●oz. softened cream cheese
- ●1 halved zucchini
- ●¼ cup shredded mozzarella cheese
- ●Garlic powder, kosher salt & black pepper
- ●½ minced jalapeno

INSTRUCTIONS

1 Adjust the oven to 4250F to preheat then grease a baking dish lightly.

2 Place the zucchini on the greased baking tray.

3 Allow to bake for 10 minutes

4 Meanwhile, take a bowl and mix the salt, mozzarella cheese, black pepper, jalapeno, cream cheese, and garlic powder

5 Remove the zucchini from oven and top them with the cheese mixture

6 Allow to bake for 8 more minutes.

7 Serve!

Nutrition Amount per serving

Calories 125, Total Fat 10.6g 14%, Saturated Fat 6.6g 33%, Cholesterol 32mg 11%, Sodium 114mg 5%, Total Carbs 4.3g 2%, Dietary Fiber 1.1g 4%, Total Sugars 1.8g, Protein 4.3g

Turkey Carrot Roll Up

Serves: 2 | Prep Time: 15 mins

INGREDIENTS

- carrot sticks
- 2 slices of turkey breasts
- 2 teaspoons yellow mustard
- 2 cheddar cheese slices
- 2 tablespoons olive oil

INSTRUCTIONS

1 Take a plate and put the turkey breast slices then sprinkle with the mustard

2 Arrange the cheddar slices then roll on the carrot sticks

3 Put a medium skillet on fire the add olive oil.

4 Sauté the turkey carrot roll ups for 3 minutes

5 Serve!

Nutrition Amount per serving

Calories 274, Total Fat 23.4g 30%, Saturated Fat 7.8g 40%, Cholesterol 43mg 15%, Sodium 660mg 29%, Total Carbs 2.5g 1%, Dietary Fiber 0.1g 1%, Total Sugars 0.1g , Protein 14.3g

Sweet & Savory Grilled Chicken

Serves: 2 | Prep Time: 25 mins

INGREDIENTS

- 1 teaspoon dry mustard
- 1 teaspoon light brown sugar
- ½ teaspoon onion powder
- ¾ pound skinless chicken breast
- Kosher salt & White pepper

INSTRUCTIONS

1 Set the grill to preheat at medium-high temperatures as you add some greasing

2 In a small bowl, add onion powder, dry mustard, salt, brown sugar, and white pepper and mix well

3 Pass the chicken meat through the mixture to coat evenly.

4 Grill the chicken for 6 minutes each side

5 Serve!

Nutrition Amount per serving

Calories 176, Total Fat 4.5g 5%, Saturated Fat 0g 0%, Cholesterol 90mg 30%, Sodium 72mg 3%, Total Carbs 2.4g 1%, Dietary Fiber 0.2g 1%, Total Sugars 1.7g, Protein 30.7g

Lemon Pepper Green Beans

Serves: 2 | Prep Time: 20 mins

INGREDIENTS

- 1 tablespoon butter
- Crushed red pepper flakes, sea salt & black pepper
- ½ pound boiled green beans
- 1 minced garlic clove
- ½ teaspoon lemon pepper seasoning

INSTRUCTIONS

1 Put a large skillet on fire to melt the butter over medium-high heat.

2 Add the lemon pepper seasoning, garlic, and red pepper flakes to fry for 1 minute then add the green beans.

3 Add black pepper and salt then cook for 5 minutes.

4 Serve!

Nutrition Amount per serving

Calories 91, Total Fat 5.8g 8%, Saturated Fat 3.6g 18%, Cholesterol 14mg 5%, Sodium 47mg 2%, Total Carbs 8.8g 3%, Dietary Fiber 4.5g 14%, Total Sugars 1.5g, Protein 2.1g

Cumin Spiced Beef Wraps

Serves: 2 | Prep Time: 30 mins

INGREDIENTS

- ¾ pound ground beef
- Salt & Black pepper, to taste
- 1½ tablespoons coconut oil
- 1 teaspoon cumin
- 4 boiled cabbage leaves

INSTRUCTIONS

1 Put a pan on fire then add coconut oil over medium heat then add the ground beef for 5 minutes.

2 Add the salt, cumin, and black pepper and cook for 5 more minutes.

3 Serve the cabbage leaves on a plate topped with the beef mixture and roll up.

4 Serve!

Nutrition Amount per serving

Calories 108, Total Fat 22g 27%, Saturated Fat 12.7g 64%, Cholesterol 151mg 51%, Sodium 190mg 8%, Total Carbs 0.6g 0%, Dietary Fiber 0.15g 0%, Total Sugars 0g, Protein 51.7g

Mahi Mahi Stew

Serves: 2 | Prep Time: 45 mins

INGREDIENTS

- 1½ tablespoons butter
- ¾ pound cubed Mahi Mahi fillets
- ½ chopped onion
- Salt & Black pepper
- ¾ cup homemade fish broth

INSTRUCTIONS

1 Sprinkle the Mahi Mahi fillets with some seasonings.

2 Put the butter in a pressure cooker to melt then add the onions

3 Cook the onions for 3 minutes then add the fish broth and mahi mahi fillets

4 Cook for 30 minutes with the lid sealed at high pressure

5 Release the pressure naturally.

6 Serve!

Nutrition Amount per serving

Calories 253, Total Fat 10.8g 14%, Saturated Fat 6.1g 32%, Cholesterol 171mg 57%, Sodium 495mg 21%, Total Carbs 2.5g 1%, Dietary Fiber 0.5g 2%, Total Sugars 1.g, Protein 34.4

Browned Butter Asparagus

Serves: 2 | Prep Time: 25 mins

INGREDIENTS

- ¼ cup sour cream
- 12 oz. green asparagus
- 1½ oz. grated parmesan cheese
- Salt & Cayenne pepper
- 1½ oz. butter

INSTRUCTIONS

1 Sprinkle the asparagus with cayenne pepper and salt

2 Put a skillet on fire then heat 1 oz. butter over medium heat

3 Sauté the asparagus for 5 minutes then transfer into a bowl

4 Put the remaining butter in skillet to heat until browned

5 Add asparagus, parmesan cheese, and sour cream.

6 Serve!

Nutrition Amount per serving

Calories 315, Total Fat 27g 36%, Saturated Fat 17.7g 89%, Cholesterol 73mg 25%, Sodium 415mg 18%, Total Carbs 8.5g 3%, Dietary Fiber 3.5g 13%, Total Sugars 3.2g , Protein 11.6g

Roasted Brussels Sprouts

Serves: 2 | Prep Time: 30 mins

INGREDIENTS

- 1 tablespoon olive oil
- 8 oz. Brussels sprouts
- ½ teaspoon dried rosemary
- 2 oz. parmesan cheese, shaved
- Salt & Black pepper

INSTRUCTIONS

1 Set the oven to 4500F to preheat then grease the baking tray with 2 tablespoons of oil.

2 Mix the Brussels sprouts with black pepper, dried rosemary, and salt then transfer to a baking tray

3 Add the parmesan cheese and olive oil on top.

4 Putin the oven to roast for 20 minutes

5 Serve!

Nutrition Amount per serving

Calories 202, Total Fat 5.3g 26%, Saturated Fat 5.5g 25%, Cholesterol 21mg 7%, Sodium 268mg 16%, Total Carbs 12g 4%, Dietary Fiber 4.5g 16%, Total Sugars 2.6g, Protein 12g

Mexican Taco Casserole

Serves: 2 | Prep Time: 35 mins

INGREDIENTS

- 1/3 cup shredded cheddar cheese
- 1/3 cup low carb salsa
- 1/3 cup cottage cheese
- ¾ pound ground beef
- ¾ tablespoon taco seasoning

INSTRUCTIONS

1 Adjust the oven to preheat at 4250F then grease a sizable baking tray lightly.

2 In a bowl, mix the ground beef and the taco seasoning

3 Add the cheddar cheese, cottage cheese, and salsa as you stir

4 Put the ground beef mixture on to the baking tray and then add the cheese mixture on top

5 Allow to bake for 25 minutes then serve warm

Nutrition Amount per serving

Calories 448, Total Fat 17.5g 23%, Saturated Fat 8.5g 42%, Cholesterol 176mg 38%, Sodium 877mg 23%, Total Carbs 6.5g 2%, Dietary Fiber 0.8g 2%, Total Sugars 2.2g, Protein 62.3g

Hamburger Patties

Serves: 2 | Prep Time: 30 mins

INGREDIENTS

- ½ egg
- 12 oz. ground beef
- 1½ oz. crumbled feta cheese
- 1 oz. butter
- Salt & Black pepper

INSTRUCTIONS

1.   In a mixing bowl, add the feta cheese, ground beef, black pepper, egg, and salt then mix to combine well.

2.   Shape the mixture into equal patties.

3.   Put a pan on fire to melt the butter.

4.   Cook the patties for 4 minutes each side on medium-low heat.

5.   Serve!

Nutrition Amount per serving

Calories 488, Total Fat 27g 36%, Saturated Fat 14.7g 74%, Cholesterol 241mg 81%, Sodium 523mg 23%, Total Carbs 2g 0%, Dietary Fiber 0g 0%, Total Sugars 2g, Protein 56.5g

Serves: 2 | Prep Time: 20 mins

INGREDIENTS

- 1 tablespoon olive oil
- ¾ pound cleaned mussels
- 1 minced garlic clove
- Salt & Black pepper
- ½ cup homemade chicken broth

INSTRUCTIONS

1.	Put a skillet on fire to heat the olive oil over medium heathen add garlic to cook for 1 minute

2.	Add the mussels and leave to cook for 5 minutes

3.	Add the seasonings and the broth as you stir gently

4.	Cook on low heat for 5 minutes with the lid covered

5.	Serve!

Nutrition Amount per serving

Calories 217, Total Fat 11.1g 14%, Saturated Fat 1.7g 9%, Cholesterol 47mg 16%, Sodium 756mg 33%, Total Carbs 6g 3%, Dietary Fiber 0g 0%

Total Sugars 0.3g, Protein 21.5g

Serves: 2 | Prep Time: 55 mins

INGREDIENTS

- ½ cup canned coconut milk
- ½ pound pork tenderloin
- 1 tablespoon Thai curry paste
- ¼ cup water
- ½ tablespoon butter

INSTRUCTIONS

1. In a mixing bowl, add the Thai curry paste, coconut milk, water, and butter then mix well
2. Take a non-stick medium skillet and put the pork meat in it.
3. Pour the coconut milk mix on the meat
4. Cook for 40 minutes while covered on medium-low heat
5. Release the pressure naturally.
6. Serve!

Nutrition Amount per serving

Calories 332, Total Fat 21.3g 27%, Saturated Fat 15.8g 79%, Cholesterol 91mg 30%, Sodium 291mg 13%, Total Carbs 4.7g 2%, Dietary Fiber 1.2g 5%, Total Sugars 2.6g, Protein 31.2g

Mediterranean Turkey Cutlets

Serves: 2 | Prep Time: 25 mins

INGREDIENTS

- 1 tablespoon olive oil
- ½ pound turkey cutlets
- ¼ cup low carb flour mix
- ½ teaspoon Greek seasoning
- ½ teaspoon turmeric powder

INSTRUCTIONS

1.   In a medium bowl, mix the turkey cutlets with turmeric powder, low carb flour mix, and Greek seasoning

2.   Put a frying pan on fire then add the oil to heat.

3.   Add the cutlets and cook for 5 minutes on each side under medium-low heat.

4.   Serve!

Nutrition Amount per serving

Calories 283, Total Fat 13.1g 17%, Saturated Fat 2g 15%, Cholesterol 85mg 29%, Sodium 481mg 21%, Total Carbs 5.6g 2%, Dietary Fiber 1.6g 6%, Total Sugars 2.4g, Protein 34.7g

DESSERTS
Cheesecake Cups

Prep + Cook Time: 10 minutes | Servings: 4

Amount per **one** serving: 205 cal., 19g fat, 5g protein & 2g carbs

INGREDIENTS
- 8 oz cream cheese, softened
- 2 oz heavy cream
- 1 tsp Stevia Glycerite
- 1 tsp Splenda
- 1 tsp vanilla flavoring (Frontier Organic)

INSTRUCTIONS
1. Combine all the ingredients.
2. Whip until a pudding consistency is achieved.
3. Divide in cups.
4. Refrigerate until served!

Strawberry Shake

Prep + Cook Time: 5 minutes | Servings: 1

Amount per **one** serving: 270 cal., 27g fat, 2.5g protein & 6.5g carbs

INGREDIENTS
- 3/4 cup coconut milk (from the carton)
- ¼ cup heavy cream
- 7 ice cubes
- 2 tbsp sugar-free strawberry Torani syrup
- ¼ tsp Xanthan Gum

INSTRUCTIONS
1. Combine all the ingredients into blender.
2. Blend for 1-2 minutes.
3. Serve!

Raspberry Pudding Surprise

Prep + Cook Time: 40 minutes | Servings: 1

Amount per **one** serving: 225 cal., 21g fat, 3g protein & 3g carbs

INGREDIENTS

- 3 tbsp chia seeds
- ½ cup unsweetened almond milk
- 1 scoop chocolate protein powder
- ¼ cup raspberries, fresh or frozen
- 1 tsp honey

INSTRUCTIONS

1. Combine the almond milk, protein powder and chia seeds together.
2. Let rest for 5 minutes before stirring.
3. Refrigerate for 30 minutes.
4. Top with raspberries.
5. Serve!

Vanilla Bean Dream

Prep + Cook Time: 35 minutes | Servings: 1

Amount per **one** serving: 205 cal., 18g fat, 7g protein & 7g carbs

INGREDIENTS

- ½ cup extra virgin coconut oil, softened
- ½ cup coconut butter, softened
- Juice of 1 lemon
- Seeds from ½ a vanilla bean

INSTRUCTIONS

1. Whisk the ingredients in an easy-to-pour cup.
2. Pour into a lined cupcake or loaf pan.
3. Refrigerate for 20 minutes. Top with lemon zest.
4. Serve!

White Chocolate Berry Cheesecake

Prep + Cook Time: 5-10 minutes | Servings: 4

Amount per **one** serving: 330 cal., 29g fat, 6g protein & 6g carbs

INGREDIENTS

- 8 oz cream cheese, softened
- 2 oz heavy cream
- ½ tsp Splenda
- 1 tsp raspberries
- 1 tbsp Da Vinci Sugar-Free syrup, white chocolate flavor

INSTRUCTIONS

1. Whip together the ingredients to a thick consistency.
2. Divide in cups.
3. Refrigerate.
4. Serve!

Coconut Pillow

Prep + Cook Time: 1-2 days | Servings: 4

Amount per **one** serving: 50 cal., 5g fat, 1g protein & 2g carbs

INGREDIENTS

- 1 can unsweetened coconut milk
- Berries of choice
- Dark chocolate

INSTRUCTIONS

1. Refrigerate the coconut milk for 24 hours.
2. Remove it from your refrigerator and whip for 2-3 minutes.
3. Fold in the berries.
4. Season with the chocolate shavings.
5. Serve!

Coffee Surprise

Prep + Cook Time: 5 minutes | Servings: 1

Amount per **one** serving: 55 cal., 45g fat, 15g protein & 3g carbs

INGREDIENTS

- 2 heaped tbsp flaxseed, ground
- 100ml cooking cream 35% fat
- ½ tsp cocoa powder, dark and unsweetened
- 1 tbsp goji berries
- Freshly brewed coffee

INSTRUCTIONS

1.   Mix together the flaxseeds, cream and cocoa and coffee.
2.   Season with goji berries.
3.   Serve!

Chocolate Cheesecake

Prep + Cook Time: 60 minutes | Servings: 4

Amount per **one** serving: 230 cal., 22g fat, 6g protein & 9g carbs

INGREDIENTS

- 4 oz cream cheese
- ½ oz heavy cream
- 1 tsp Stevia Glycerite
- 1 tsp Splenda
- 1 oz Enjoy Life mini chocolate chips

INSTRUCTIONS

1.   Combine all the ingredients except the chocolate to a thick consistency.
2.   Fold in the chocolate chips.
3.   Refrigerate in serving cups.
4.   Serve!

Almond Crusty

Prep + Cook Time: 60 minutes | Servings: 4

Amount per **one** serving: 190 cal., 18g fat, 8g protein & 5g carbs

INGREDIENTS

- 1 cup keto almond flour
- 4 tsp melted butter
- 2 large eggs
- ½ tsp salt

INSTRUCTIONS

1. Mix together the almond flour and butter.
2. Add in the eggs and salt and combine well to form a dough ball.
3. Place the dough between two pieces of parchment paper. Roll out to 10" by 16" and ¼ inch thick.
4. Bake for 30 minutes at 350°F, or until golden brown.
5. Serve!

Chocolate Peanut Butter Cups

Prep + Cook Time: 70 minutes | Servings: 2

Amount per **one** serving: 175 cal., 17g fat, 2g protein & 12g carbs

INGREDIENTS

- 1 stick unsalted butter
- 1 oz / 1 cube unsweetened chocolate
- 5 packets Stevia in the Raw
- 1 tbsp heavy cream
- 4 tbsp peanut butter

INSTRUCTIONS

1. In a microwave, melt the butter and chocolate.
2. Add the Stevia.
3. Stir in the cream and peanut butter.
4. Line the muffin tins. Fill the muffin cups.
5. Freeze for 60 minutes.
6. Serve!

Macaroons Bites

Prep + Cook Time: 30 minutes | Servings: 2

Amount per **one** serving: 125 cal., 12g fat, 2g protein & 5g carbs

INGREDIENTS

- 4 egg whites
- ½ tsp vanilla
- ½ tsp EZ-Sweet (or equivalent of 1 cup artificial sweetener)
- 4½ tsp water
- 1 cup unsweetened coconut

INSTRUCTIONS

1. Preheat your oven to 375°F/190°C.
2. Combine the egg whites, liquids and coconut.
3. Put into the oven and reduce the heat to 325°F/160°C.
4. Bake for 15 minutes.
5. Serve!

Choco-berry Fudge Sauce

Prep + Cook Time: 30 minutes | Servings: 2

Amount per **one** serving: 155 cal., 15g fat, 2g protein & 4g carbs

INGREDIENTS

- 4 oz cream cheese, softened
- 1-3.5 oz 90% chocolate Lindt bar, chopped
- ¼ cup powdered erythritol
- ¼ cup heavy cream
- 1 tbsp Monin sugar-free raspberry syrup

INSTRUCTIONS

1. In a large skillet, melt together the cream cheese and chocolate.
2. Stir in the sweetener.
3. Remove from the heat and allow to cool.
4. Once cool, mix in the cream and syrup.
5. Serve!

Choco-Coconut Pudding

Prep + Cook Time: 65 minutes | Servings: 1

Amount per **one** serving: 225 cal., 23g fat, 4g protein & 5g carbs

INGREDIENTS

- 1 cup coconut milk
- 2 tbsp cacao powder or organic cocoa
- ½ tsp Stevia powder extract or 2 tbsp honey/maple syrup
- ½ tbsp quality gelatin
- 1 tbsp water

INSTRUCTIONS

1.   On a medium heat, combine the coconut milk, cocoa and sweetener.
2.   In a separate bowl, mix in the gelatin and water.
3.   Add to the pan and stir until fully dissolved.
4.   Pour into small dishes and refrigerate for 1 hour.
5.   Serve!

Strawberry Frozen Dessert

Prep + Cook Time: 45 minutes | Servings: 1

Amount per **one** serving: 85 cal., 5g fat, 2g protein & 5g carbs

INGREDIENTS

- ½ cup sugar-free strawberry preserves
- ½ cup Stevia in the Raw or Splenda
- 2 cups Fage Total 0% Greek Yogurt
- Ice cream maker

INSTRUCTIONS

1.   In a food processor, purée the strawberries. Add the strawberry preserves.
2.   Add the Greek yogurt and fully mix.
3.   Put into the ice cream maker for 25-30 minute.
4.   Serve!

Berry Layer Cake

Prep + Cook Time: 8 minutes | Servings: 1

Amount per **one** serving: 450 cal., 35g fat, 12g protein & 5g carbs

INGREDIENTS

- ¼ lemon pound cake
- ¼ cup whipping cream
- ½ tsp Truvia
- 1/8 tsp orange flavor
- 1 cup of mixed berries

INSTRUCTIONS

1. Using a sharp knife, divide the lemon cake into small cubes.
2. Dice the strawberries.
3. Combine the whipping cream, Truvia, and orange flavor.
4. Layer the fruit, cake and cream in a glass.
5. Serve!

Chocolate Pudding

Prep + Cook Time: 50 minutes | Servings: 1

Amount per **one** serving: 430 cal., 42g fat, 4g protein & 5g carbs

INGREDIENTS

- 3 tbsp chia seeds
- 1 cup unsweetened almond milk
- 1 scoop cocoa powder
- ¼ cup fresh raspberries
- ½ tsp keto friendly honey

INSTRUCTIONS

1. Mix together all of the ingredients in a large bowl.
2. Let rest for 15 minutes but stir half way through.
3. Stir again and refrigerate for 30 minutes. Garnish with raspberries.
4. Serve!

Cranberry Cream Surprise

Prep + Cook Time: 30 minutes | Servings: 2

Amount per **one** serving: 333 cal., 24g fat, 8g protein & 4g carbs

INGREDIENTS

- 1 cup mashed cranberries
- ½ cup Confectioner's Style Swerve
- 2 tsp natural cherry flavoring
- 2 tsp natural rum flavoring
- 1 cup organic heavy cream

INSTRUCTIONS

1. Combine the mashed cranberries, sweetener, cherry and rum flavorings.
2. Cover and refrigerate for 20 minutes.
3. Whip the heavy cream until soft peaks form.
4. Layer the whipped cream and cranberry mixture.
5. Top with fresh cranberries, mint leaves or grated dark chocolate.
6. Serve!

APPENDIX : RECIPES INDEX

Lightning Source UK Ltd.
Milton Keynes UK
UKHW051857290722
406599UK00005B/326